Peaceful Heart, Healthy Body

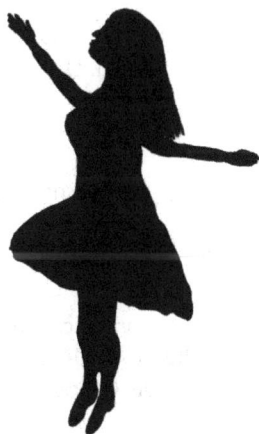

Michelle Watson

Peaceful Hearth, Healthy Body

Cover Designer: Michelle Watson

ISBN: 978-0-9996054-4-8

Printed in the United States of America

Topflight Communication, Inc.
PO Box 390426
Snellville, GA 30039
www.topflightcommunication.com

This book is dedicated to

Lee Watson
My husband
in riches and in lack,
in sickness and in health.
You have always stood beside me,
no matter the pain or the illness.
I love you and appreciate you
more than I can say.

Introduction

Proverbs 14:30 says, "A peaceful heart leads to a healthy body." I have certainly found this to be true. It can be an obvious answer when bitterness and resentment have caused physical sickness and pain. But, even when there is truly something medically wrong that causes physical ailments, maintaining a peaceful heart throughout the situation can help the body heal or become healthy.

My life of more than 30 years of pain started when I was eight years old. That was when the headaches started. The migraines continued for years, followed by all kinds of aches and pains throughout my body. Before I even turned 40, I often told people I felt like I was 90—and I wasn't exaggerating!

As I looked to many different methods for healing, I came to know this one thing—God heals. Sometimes, spiritual issues such as bitterness lead to physical ailments that are healed instantly after forgiving the offending party. Other times, doctors remove foreign masses or other invaders from our bodies, but it is God who guides the surgeon's hand. And still other times, the healing may come from modern medicines, natural remedies, or lifestyle changes.

Not all physical problems are caused by spiritual problems. But, when there is no medical explanation, as you will often read about in my story, a peaceful heart does lead to a healthy body. When doctors could not give me an accurate diagnosis, I learned quickly to seek God for the answer. He can *always* tell the doctors or me what needs to be done to reach my healing.

This memoir chronicles my personal journey to health. The stories are in chronological order, although they each span different time periods, and often overlap each other. The conversations are as accurate as I remember, though they are often condensed. It made the story flow more smoothly to combine several conversations into one or two. Facts and dates have been reconstructed from my memory, social media post histories, and available medical records. The names of all my doctors and health practitioners have been changed. I had too many to remember them all, but they are all important. I also changed their names because I went through a period of time in which I saw a number of doctors who were very unhelpful. They weren't particularly bad doctors. They may help many of their patients; they just did not help me, and I don't want to disparage any of their reputations.

My journey to health is not complete. I am only 45 as of this publication, so I know I have a lot of life left to experience. I am in an aging body bound to an Earth that is still suffering from man's first decision to sin. I am otherwise healthy because I learned to accept God's gift of peace through any trial or circumstance. I am thankful for the chance to write about the different physical ailments I have been healed from, knowing it will build my faith and yours to remain healthy and healed.

I hope that in each chapter you will find something that relates to your own situation. Let God show you what form of healing is right for you. Pray He gives you and your health providers wisdom. He is always faithful to answer, sometimes in creative ways that you might have never considered.

May God bless you with a *Peaceful Heart, Healthy Body*.

Contributing Factors

When I was eight years old, my mother, brother, and I were standing in the grocery store in Enid, Oklahoma. It was like any other shopping trip, except for one small incident. A store employee on the next aisle was stocking the top shelf. He pushed something back too hard and too far, and it knocked a jelly jar over the edge and onto my head.

There wasn't a need for stitches; the jar didn't break until it hit the floor. I did get a knot on my head and, according to my mom, this was the trigger that started my headaches.

I don't know how often the headaches came. I do know they occurred quite often and that, after several months to a year, my mom was desperate to ease my pain. I had a nauseating headache one night at church. We were hosting a guest preacher who was praying for people to be healed. My mom told him about my headaches and how the jar hitting my head had seemed to be the starting point. She asked him to pray for me. He came over to where I was lying on the pew, laid his hands on me, and prayed.

"Lord, heal this child of these headaches. Let them be gone in the name of Jesus."

Looking at me, he asked, "Are you feeling better?"

"No, it still hurts."

Laying hands on my head again, he prayed, "We command the headache to go. Be healed."

I opened my eyes and looked at him again. *Why is he so close to my face?*

"Does your head still hurt?"

"Yes," I barely nodded.

"Father, we know You are the Healer and You want this child to be made well. We ask that You touch her now and loose these headaches from her body in Jesus' name."

This is boring. And why does he have to be so close? He makes funny faces when he prays like that.

He asked the inevitable question again, "Are you feeling better now?"

"Yes, it doesn't hurt anymore," I lied.

I had had enough. The man wasn't scary; I wasn't afraid of him or uneasy at his presence. But, because he had gotten down to where I was, he was in my face, and I wanted him gone. I was bored with the repeated process and just wanted to be left alone. Of course he and everyone else in the church that night rejoiced that the headaches were gone, that I was healed. Except, the headaches weren't really gone and I wasn't really healed.

By the time I was in ninth grade, the headaches came so often and were so painful that my mom got desperate to find a root cause for my headaches. She was a single mother of three. We had everything we needed. She saw to that, but, as could be expected, we still lived rather simply. Although our needs were met, there wasn't any money to waste or spend frivolously.

My mom's quest to find a cure for my headaches started with a late-night visit to the hospital. I had a headache so bad that night I could barely move. Our apartment was a small rectangle. The front door opened to a modest living room. The dining area and kitchen, on the back side of the door, were together the same size as the living room. The hallway that led to the single bathroom and three bedrooms was very short, probably about seven feet. But that night, as I crawled to my bedroom, that hallway may as well have been a mile long.

It was the worst headache I had experienced in my life up to that point. My mom helped me to the car and then drove me to the emergency room. I don't remember the hospital waiting room or walking down the hall as the nurse escorted us back. I do remember what came next, though. Especially the doctor. He was not happy with me at all, and it was enough to traumatize any child.

I lay on the gurney as instructed. The doctor and all the medical equipment of an emergency room bed were so close that, for the first time that I remember, I actually felt oppression in the air. The more he asked me about my headache, the worse I felt. Not just because I was in pain, but because the doctor and all the equipment that surrounded the bed gave me a slight feeling of claustrophobia. Just as with the man who had prayed for me so many years before, I just wanted the doctor out of my face and to get myself out of there as quickly as possible.

At first, the doctor was understanding, "Okay, Michelle, I am going to give you a shot of morphine. Just relax."

He jiggled my buttock. "Relax this muscle," he repeated.

I was in a lot of pain, and I hated getting shots. My childhood pediatrician gave me an antibiotic shot nearly every time I had to see him. I had developed a permanent aversion to shots in the behind. I couldn't relax. I involuntarily tensed up.

This made the doctor quite angry—and it would later aggravate me, too.

"Michelle, I told you to relax. You tensed up. Look there, you bent the needle. Now, I have to give you another shot with another needle. Make sure you relax this time."

He walked around to the other side of the bed and jiggled the other buttock. This time it worked. I didn't tense up, and when it was all over, the headache was gone. My pain, however, was far from over.

Over the next 24-48 hours, I developed two large bruises, the largest I have ever seen. They were on each side of my behind, right where the doctor had put the injections. What's worse is that the shots caused a great amount of pain in the muscles. It hurt to walk and I couldn't sit back in my desk at school, or anywhere else, for that matter. At home, I crawled around as much as I could to keep from walking, but at school I somehow muddled through.

That trip to the ER was more than my mom could take. She tried all the more to find out the cause of my headaches.

She took me to a doctor who tested me for diabetes. I didn't have it. Another doctor said I needed eyeglasses for close-up work. I was to wear them at school and for "close-up" work, but I didn't need them any other time. Actually, it turned out I didn't need them at all. They gave me a different kind of headache from sitting so heavily on my nose, and they made the words on the page blurry. I figured if my vision was not blurry without glasses, and only blurry when I wore them, I should just not wear the glasses. So, I decided not to. I wonder now how much it cost my mom to buy those glasses. I feel bad for simply deciding not to wear them instead of going back to the doctor for an improved prescription. No one in my immediate family had worn glasses up to that point, so none of us really knew anything about them or how optical prescriptions worked.

The most expensive and time-consuming diagnosis came when my mom took me to the orthodontist. He said I had temporomandibular joint disorder (TMJ, or TMD as it is called today), and that I needed braces. My current dentist and orthodontist both tell me that I could get braces again if I want straighter teeth, but they won't improve anything. They assure me braces will not stop TMD, keep me from grinding my teeth, or even improve my bite, and that they didn't really help all those years ago. Doctors had just been taught they would, and they believed it. I wish, though, that first orthodontist had not been so sure braces would stop my headaches. He might have saved my mom a lot of money, because the headaches kept coming for many more years.

When I was 23, I began to see some hope for relief. When our pastor's wife died, he asked the church to pray and fast with him 40 days. He wanted clear direction from God on what he and the church should do next. I had never fasted, and I had been warned not to do a full 40-day fast if I had no experience with shorter ones. I had recently been discussing the dangers of caffeine with a friend of mine. I recalled how I had never gotten a headache when I was pregnant, and the one thing I abstained from during my pregnancy was caffeine. So, I decided that while the rest of the church fasted, I would give up caffeine and see what happened. The entire time I fasted, I did not get one headache. I did drink some Dr. Pepper at the end of the fast to see what happened, and as I expected, I got a terrible migraine.

I gave up caffeine permanently from that moment. I had never been one to rely on caffeine for energy, so it was easier for me than it is for most people. Giving up the taste of Dr. Pepper did take some getting used to, but I quickly learned to enjoy Sprite and root beer. Giving up sweet tea was a little more difficult. Even though I never could tell the difference in taste between decaffeinated coffee and regular, I could sure tell the difference between decaffeinated iced tea and regular iced tea.

Giving up tea altogether was much easier than getting used to the taste of decaffeinated.

Once I returned to a normal diet (sans caffeine), the headaches continued to come. They came less frequently, but they were more painful and debilitating than they had ever been. I would get nauseated and couldn't stand sound or light. I couldn't even stand closing my eyes because doing so made the pressure in my head so much worse.

I remember one night I was supposed to go to church for an evening service after work. My friend Missy had watched my daughter, Arienne, for me that day and was going to bring her to me at church. I couldn't get there, though. I took a co-worker home and ended up staying at her house until I felt well enough to drive. I lay on one of her boys' beds until I felt up to rising, but even then I felt horribly sick. Somehow, I finally mustered the resolve to get to the church, pick up my Arienne, and drive home.

Another time I was leaving Bible study at Missy's house. I had a headache when I left, but was sure I could make it home. Had I known just how bad the headache really was, I probably would have asked Missy if I could stay the night. But when you are sick, all you want is your own bed. I got in my car and headed home. I nearly didn't make it. I was so nauseated I was sure I was going to throw up. I stopped three times during the 20-minute drive home.

The first stop was on the side of the road, where I nearly vomited, but somehow I avoided it. The second time was in an empty church parking lot. It was late enough that I knew no one was there, and I just hoped to rest enough to gain the strength to get home. When I made the third stop, I was probably two minutes from home. I just couldn't make it another inch. I pulled into a fire station parking lot, half hoping one of the men would come out to check on me, but no one did. I rested as much as I could (it's hard to rest when you're sick and you are worried about your young child being in the car with you). Finally, I sat up with enough strength to make it home. I went to bed, and awoke the next morning without so much as a hint of the headache from the night before. My headaches' going was becoming as mysterious as their coming.

About this time, it began to dawn on me that perhaps caffeine was not the source of my headaches after all. I began to hear others talk about triggers and how high blood pressure could be the problem, since caffeine was at least one apparent trigger. It definitely increases your blood pressure. In fact, one health food store employee flat-out told me that my sensitivity to caffeine could be a sign that I would have high blood pressure later in life. I refused to accept his negative prognosis, and I can thankfully say he was wrong. To this day I have never had high blood pressure, not even when I was in the middle of some of the worst headaches of my life.

No, there had to be something else, I was sure. Whether it was something I was eating or some other unknown reason, I was determined I would find the source of my headaches. So, I talked to people. I discussed what friends and others knew about migraine triggers. I tried eliminating every food I heard about being a "known" trigger. I found out about MSG from my boss, Steve.

"A man at the health food store told me that getting a migraine from caffeine could be a sign I will have high blood pressure someday," I told Steve in a casual conversation.

"That's possible."

"I don't know, though. There is one restaurant I like, but I get a headache every time I get there. It's BD's Mongolian BBQ."

"If it's every time, it could be the food. It's Oriental food, right?"

"Yeah, well, you make your own. All the food is on different bars. You go to the meat bar and get your meat, then to the vegetable bar, and then you put all the spices on it that you want. You take it to the grill and they fry it, put it in a clean bowl, and give it back to you."

"But, I'm saying, if it's Oriental, it could have MSG. If you have blood pressure issues, MSG can make them worse."

"Oh. Well, I don't have high blood pressure, but it's worth a try. I have eaten there three times and got a headache every time."

I did some online research on BD's and found out they had a list of foods that contained MSG. All I had to do was ask for it. The next time I ate at BD's, I asked for the list and I diligently avoided everything on the list. To my surprise, and great joy, I also avoided the usual headache.

Over the years, by trial and error, I learned that anything meant to increase one's energy or metabolism can be a trigger for migraines. I added vitamin B (all of them), chromium picolinate, MSG, ginseng, and more, to the list of foods and ingredients to be eliminated from my diet. Avoiding all these things did help—some. I could avoid one trigger, and thus the resulting headache, for a time. But, over time, even if I never ate any one food again, the headaches returned as strong as, or stronger than, before.

The headaches just kept coming. I was *sure* I was missing some rare trigger and that learning to avoid it was the answer.

God had a better answer.

The Migraine Miracle

I am grateful for the miracle that finally cured my recurrent migraines, even if the road was a long and crooked one. In fact, it might be the difficult journey that makes the victory so sweet.

When you suffer from any kind of headache, even frequent ones, it is hard to find a doctor who will do anything significant for you. Many doctors are reluctant to admit a patient has migraines if the symptoms don't fit a specific clinical definition they think it should. If you see six different doctors, you will get six different diagnoses. I learned to be my own advocate and to be persistent. It helped with my headaches, but these skills served me well later in life, too.

I remember the first time I was notably irritated with a doctor. It was time for my annual gynecology appointment. Like always, the paperwork and her questions included an inquiry into my medical history, including headaches. I had such a long history of headaches I naturally selected "yes" on the form.

"You get headaches?" asked Dr. Cobb.

"Yes."

"How frequently?"

"Several times a month, sometimes more," I said, trying to give her a reasonable estimate.

"What kind of headaches are they?" she asked.

I had not received an official diagnosis up to that point, so I guessed, "I think they are migraines."

"Where do they hurt?"

I wish doctors knew how hard it is to answer that question when you aren't currently suffering, I thought as I told her the best I could how badly the front of my head and temples hurt at their worst.

"Do you throw up?"

"No, but I get nauseated."

"But you don't throw up."

"Not usually. Usually I just feel like I'm going to."

"If you aren't throwing up, they aren't migraines. They are sinus headaches."

I tried to get her to understand just how nauseated I got. I am talking, sit-on-the-floor-and-grab-the-great-ceramic-bowl-like-you-have-a-hangover kind of nauseated.

She didn't listen. She only got angrier and surer in her conviction, "If you aren't throwing up, they can't *possibly* be migraines."

I left Dr. Cobb's office without any help, and without hope that relief would ever come.

On September 11, 2001 I decided to rule out the possibility that my headaches could be caused by a need for glasses. When you have recurring headaches, an eye exam is one of the first things many friends and doctors recommend. It was a day I will never forget.

After the initial exam, Dr. Vann put the dilation drops in my eyes.

"The drops will take a few minutes," he said. "You can go out and walk around Walmart for ten minutes if you like, or you can sit and wait in the lobby."

"Okay. I think I will walk around a bit."

I didn't need anything in the store, so I just wandered around. When I got to the electronics department, President George W. Bush was addressing the nation after two planes had crashed into the twin towers in New York City. I had misunderstood, though. I thought only one tower was hit.

I went back to the doctor's office and sat in his lobby until he was ready for me. The radio was on, and of course the news continued to broadcast updates of the day's events.

"The two towers of the World Trade Center have collapsed," I heard the announcer say.

I occasionally talk out loud to a waiting room of strange people. The shock of the news made this rare habit much more likely to occur.

I perked up and looked around the room, "*Two* towers? I thought it was only one."

I shrunk back into my seat as I felt the weight of their stares. No one else in the room was nearly as alarmed as I was and they just looked blankly at me, like they had not even heard the radio announcer. I didn't say anything else as long as we all sat there, but I couldn't help wondering, *Why don't they care?*

It was my turn to return to the doctor's exam room. I was thankful Dr. Vann finished quickly. I was anxious to get home.

"You don't need glasses. Your vision is nearly perfect."

I was sure I knew that, but I was glad to have a doctor's confirmation. I got in the car to drive home and turned on the radio.

The news continued, "We now have word that a third plane crashed into the Pentagon in Washington, DC."

My husband, Lee, was still in the Air Force at the time. I knew that if the attacks continued, he would need to be on high alert.

They might call him in, or even send him to war. All I could think about was getting home, to him, and to the news on the TV.

I pulled in the driveway and rushed in the door to wake Lee. He was asleep because, as with the majority of our marriage, he worked the graveyard shift.

I jumped on the bed, "Get up! America is being attacked and you are sleeping through the whole thing!"

He woke up enough to understand the need to follow me into the living room. We turned on the television and learned of the fourth plane being taken down in a field in Pennsylvania, its target still unknown at that time.

It took a while to all sink in. Sometimes today, even in remembering it so vividly, it seems surreal the way the events unfolded as I heard an update about a plane-turned-torpedo each time I tuned into the news. It was a bittersweet day. I was grateful I didn't need glasses, but brokenhearted and angry for our country.

I wasn't sure where I would turn next to get medical help with my headaches. An answer came without much trouble after a couple of emergency trips to the doctor. The doctor I was seeing by this time had an after-hours minor emergency clinic. Each doctor in the building was independent, but they all rotated serving after hours.

My friend Mary took me to the after-hours clinic that night and sat with Arienne in the waiting room. When the nurse called me back, I learned I would have the honor of being treated by Cassidy, my doctor's physician's assistant. Cassidy asked me some questions and gave me an IV before sending me home. Mary and Arienne eventually came back to my room and waited with me the whole time.

That was when the real trouble started. Mary and I, in our rush to get my pain diagnosed and stopped, did not make sure I had everything I needed. I had forgotten my house key! I was in too much pain to think. Mary called her son and asked him if he could come over and help us get in. Michael came, but our house, with its tight-frame windows, was not easy to break into. You can't just slide up a trailer window. So, Michael tried to break the window in our back door. It would not give way. He succeeded in cracking the frame around the glass pane, but the glass never did break.

I had to do the one thing left—find a locksmith. I don't know how I got the number, but I called someone who came right over, and unlocked my house for us. I am thankful Mary was there that night. I was miserable with both a headache and nausea.

The second time I went to the clinic and saw Cassidy, it was in the regular-hours office. She surprised me when she let me know she was a little tired of seeing me for the same thing. To this day, I believe it was by God's providence that I saw the same doctor both times I went in with a headache. When some doctors get tired of seeing a patient for the same thing, they make the patient feel embarrassed or burdensome. Not Cassidy. She made me feel like she wanted me to finally have an answer—and she didn't even know my whole story.

"You've been in here with a headache pretty often, haven't you," Cassidy asked.

I shrugged, "Yeah, I guess I have." I didn't mean to take it so casually, but two times in her office did not seem to me to be "pretty often." In my head, I was trying to think back if maybe I had seen her more times for my headaches and I just didn't remember.

"Well, I am going to send you to a neurologist. I think you need to find out why you are getting these headaches and get some help."

"Okay," I tried to sound cheerful and show as much gratitude as I could muster in spite of the pain. I really was grateful that after what was now 24 years of headaches I was about to get the help I needed.

The neurologist, Dr. Lacy, was amazing. Her office was bright and airy, and in a newly constructed medical building. The walls were decorated with large black and white canvas prints of photos of her newborn twins. But, it was Dr. Lacy's perkiness and eagerness to serve that I remember most.

I shared with Dr. Lacy some of the things I had been told. Like many other doctors I have encountered over the years, she rolled her eyes in disgust when I told her of the doctor who had once said I "couldn't possibly" have migraines. This gave me an instant love for her, to say the least.

"I am going to order a CAT scan. That is the first thing we need to do, just to rule out any tumors or other conditions."

"Okay. That sounds good."

"In the meantime, I am going to prescribe Imitrex. You must take it at the first onset of the migraine. If you wait too long to take it, it won't do much good. Is there anything else you take that helps when you get a headache?"

"Well, Tylenol makes me throw up, but Darvocet helps. I can't take codeine or Percocet because they just give me a headache. In fact, I can time the headache to start exactly 24 hours later."

"Okay, then I am going to give you Darvocet just in case you get a headache and the Imitrex doesn't stop it."

"Great. Thank you."

Up to this point, I had been through a bone scan and possibly an MRI. I had been through various types of x-rays, too. One x-ray I had when I was very young was done in a machine I stepped into and it turned me sideways. At least that is what I remember, but the memories of a child are often misunderstood impressions.

The CAT scan was different from all other machines and tests, though. I looked at the "machine," which was a large black loop with a rainbow of lights going around it. In spite of its small size, it brought to mind a loop that a circus rider or a daredevil might drive around. I lay on the table with my head positioned under the lighted ring and waited for the test to finish.

The results were hopeful, or not, depending on how you look at it.

Dr. Lacy gave me the news, "Well, the good news is your results are clear. You don't have any tumors or other disorders."

"That's good," came my hope-filled reply.

"Have the headaches changed or gotten better?"

"I am getting one almost every day. The Imitrex and Darvocet help. They are coming so frequently, though, I just want them to stop."

"Okay, well, we are going to try a few more things. I am going to start with a round of steroids. Often when headaches come in clusters like this, a good dose of steroids will help knock out whatever is in your system that is causing them."

I returned to see Dr. Lacy after I finished the steroids. They hadn't helped. In fact, the frequency of my headaches had only increased to the point that I was getting one every day. Dr. Lacy was still sure she had an answer and we would get to it, one way or another.

Dr. Lacy started with a newly approved medication, "I am going to prescribe Topamax and see how you do on that."

"Oh, I have seen that advertised on TV a lot lately," I said, a little relieved to hear her mention something I had at least a little familiarity with.

She proceeded to explain to me how it was originally created as a neurological medication. In the trial studies, it came to light that, among other things, Topamax prevented migraines. Once they obtained FDA approval to make the claim as a migraine preventative, the makers advertised in all the women's magazines. It didn't take long for its popularity to skyrocket.

Topamax certainly did the job it claimed it would, but not without some unmanageable side effects.

"Did the Topamax help?" Dr. Lacy asked.

"Oh, it works great. I love that I can have caffeine again without getting a headache. I still can't take Vitamin B, but I can drink sweet tea again!"

"Well, that's good," she said as we laughed together.

"But, there are side effects I can't handle. My fingertips tingle and go numb. I can't type or play my flute. And, my face goes numb from the bottom of my chin to the tip of my nose, including my lips and the tip of my tongue."

"That's not so good. Other than that you like it, though, right?"

"Yes, other than the numbness I love it. But I can't take it if I can't even do my job."

"No, you can't," Dr. Lacy agreed. "Okay. I'm going to try a different medicine in the same class. Zonegran is another anti-seizure medication, but it has been around a lot longer. It shouldn't have the same side effects."

"Great. Let's try it."

I was thrilled that Zonegran was everything Dr. Lacy promised it would be. Unlike with Topamax, I had to return to being caffeine-free. But, the headaches quit coming, and I didn't have the tingling and numbness I had with Topamax. Dr. Lacy kept me on Darvocet for those occasions when I still got a headache.

I would have loved to continue seeing Dr. Lacy, but my husband was soon transferred from North Carolina to New Jersey. I didn't want to go through the horrible process of convincing a new doctor I needed a local neurologist, so I decided not to even try. I took myself off the Zonegran and suffered through the return of the migraines. I am saddened looking back that this meant my family also suffered with me, but it was the catalyst that spurred me on to earnestly pray one more time for healing.

As I lay in bed one Saturday night, suffering from the worst headache I'd had in two years, I prayed. I don't remember if it was a prayer of faith or desperation. I do remember what I prayed.

"Father God," I sounded so weak, even to myself. "I can't keep getting these headaches. Constantly being sick is not a good testimony to my husband of who You are. I pray these headaches would start to gradually lessen to the point that I no longer get them, and it would serve as a testimony to my husband of Your healing power."

The next morning I went to church, determined I was going to get prayer and that these headaches were going to stop once and for all. I spoke first with the pastor. He asked Elder Danita to come over and pray for me. To my amazement, she prayed almost exactly what I had prayed, including a request that the headaches would lessen until I just didn't get them anymore. It was like she was in the room with me the night before!

To God be the glory that from that moment until this, I have not had a single migraine. Nearly 30 years of severe headaches just stopped. I do get an occasional headache, usually associated with something I have done or eaten, or with my monthly cycle. But, never again have I gotten the kind of debilitating headache that once made me crawl on the floor, brought me to my knees in the bathroom, or left me begging for prescription pain medications.

An update to this story has occurred since I started writing this book: I have been drinking sweet tea again with no ill effects. Not even a hint of a headache.

When God heals, His healing is complete—through and through!

Rooting Out Bitterness

I was 17 years old when I got pregnant in 1991. I was a senior in high school, and it turned my world upside down. It also led to eight years of pain, and my discovery of how spiritual healing can bring physical healing.

I jokingly said to my boyfriend, "You know, I *might* be pregnant."

I didn't even know if I was, and had no real reason for saying something like that. Up to that point, I didn't have any symptoms. Not even the most common one—a late cycle. No matter why I said it, I am glad I did, because I never really saw him again. I was actually happy to have him out of our lives if that was going to be his reaction. Oh, sure, like most girls would, I had fun daydreaming of our becoming a loving family, of his stepping up and taking responsibility.

But, I was not so naïve as to believe we would happily grow old together. I knew what kind of person he was. He drank and did drugs, and rumor had it that he dealt drugs for his dad. I knew that if he did not want anything to do with us I would move on without him and his troublesome family. I had fought to keep guys in my life before, but this was different somehow. I didn't chase him down and try to keep him because I just couldn't bring myself to do it. Someone later told me of another girl he got pregnant after he and I broke up. The story was that he was staying with her to prevent her going after him for child support. That was *not* a hassle I needed or wanted, and I knew my baby girl didn't, so I let him walk out of our lives with no further contact.

Shortly after my Arienne was born, I developed pain on the left side of my body—my back hip, otherwise known as the gluteus medius, to be exact. There didn't seem to be a cause for the pain. The doctor sent me to physical therapy. It was my first time ever seeing a physical therapist, so I had no idea what to expect. I wanted it to work out well, but our relationship didn't last long.

At my first appointment Joan asked about my lifestyle and what I did for a living. I told her about my newborn baby and my receptionist job. Joan took the time to educate me on how these two things affected my back.

Joan stood in front of me as I sat in a chair, and explained, "When you hold something in front of you, the weight on your back is three times more than the weight of the object you are holding."

"Oh. Really?" This was news to me. I just listened.

"Next," she said, "when you are sitting, you are really bending over."

Joan demonstrated what she meant. She stood up, bent over, and then bent her knees. She was showing me that whether you stand up and bend over or sit down for eight hours a day, your back is in the same position. Your lower back will react with the same pain, stiffness, and weakness when you sit for long periods as it would if you bent forward for that same period of time.

It was really eye-opening, but there was not much I could do about it. My job was my job. I didn't know what I could do about my work environment. The pain had started at least a year prior, when I was still working at a drugstore where I was standing on my feet all day. So, I was not as thoroughly convinced as Joan was that sitting was the source of my problem.

Joan finished her initial assessment and lecture. She had me do some exercises and sent me home with a daily routine similar to what my doctor had given me. In addition to this, my bosses tried to help as much as they could, but the study and promotion of ergonomics were still quite new. In 1993 people did not just scour the internet for information. It's funny how things changed in just two short years, and suddenly everything you ever wanted to know was online by 1995.

The company where I worked, CDI Corporation, purchased a back brace I could use when I was standing at the filing cabinet. I tried to wear sneakers to and from the office while I rode the bus and train to work. The adjustment my back and hips made when switching from high heels back to sneakers at the end of the work day only aggravated the pain. It was easier to wear my heels all day, no matter how bad that was for my back. In spite of everything I tried, the pain continued, and I grew weary of hoping for improvement.

"We are going to try something different today," Joan said on what I think was my fourth visit. "Let's get her on the ultrasound table," she instructed her assistant.

The ultrasound seemed pointless to me, but since I didn't know anything about physical therapy or my condition at the time, I went along with anything Joan recommended. I think, though, that my frustration at my lack of improvement must have been easily recognizable.

"Talk to me. What's going on," Joan asked.

"Nothing," I said. "I just don't think I belong here."

"If you don't think you need to be here, why are you here?"

I sat in stunned silence. I didn't know what to say. I was there because I trusted my doctor and most other medical professionals, and if they said it was what I needed, I was at least willing to try it.

Joan's ire rose as she almost shrieked, "Seriously. If you don't think you need to be here, *why* are you here?"

She was the first medical professional to get angry when I dared to question her expertise or authority. Unfortunately, she wouldn't be the last. I learned in time to stand up to them and give an answer for my opinion, but I was quite young at only 19 years old. So, I took Joan's question, and her anger, to heart. I didn't return. I never will know if staying in therapy would have helped, but as I think about what I endured over the next six to seven years, I am convinced that nothing Joan would have done for me would have made much difference.

Yes, you read that right—the pain continued for about seven years after I last saw Joan, for a total of eight years. I tried everything during that time. I went to the gym. I visited doctors occasionally when the pain was unbearable. I did the physical therapy exercises Joan and the doctors gave me. I took pain medications and muscle relaxers. I tried hot baths. Nothing helped for eight years. The one bone scan a doctor had ordered revealed no source of the pain. I was convinced I was doomed to live with the pain the rest of my life.

In November 1995 I married Lee Watson. Lee and I had met while I was pregnant, and we wed when my Arienne was three. He had come to accept my pain as much as I had, and he cared for me through all of it. It makes me sad to think about how much my child was taking care of the cooking by the time she was eight. I was there to make sure she was safe when she went in the kitchen, and a lot of times she simply helped her father cook. They especially enjoyed making hamburgers together. He put every seasoning in the cabinet into the mix, and she had fun squishing her hands in the meat—something I dislike to this day, so I am glad she enjoyed it. I could get around enough to make sure she was clothed, bathed, and fed well. But, a lot of my time at home was spent lying on the couch in pain, wishing the pain pills would work.

I tried to be more physically active, knowing that too much inactivity was not good for my back. I started a job working for a fire and smoke damage restoration company. The stress on my back was hard, but it was bearable until I quit working at the end of the day. As long as I kept moving I seemed to be okay. It was only after I got home from a job site and sat down that the pain and stiffness were so strong I could barely stand back up.

I did learn that if I exercised that buttock muscle after work, in spite of how tired or sore I was, I could fatigue the muscle to such a point of weakness that it didn't hurt as much. I was willing to try anything. I even joined the dance ministry because I believed God told me to use dance as a form of spiritual warfare.

Our pastor, Emory Goodman, had been preaching on Joshua 7 and 8. Chapter 7 tells us the nation of Israel had gone to fight the city of Ai. God's people were dumbfounded because their enemy was able to simply run them off. Later in the chapter, we read that Achan's sin was the reason for their defeat. Because he had disobeyed and kept forbidden spoils of war, the entire nation of Israel paid the price. In Chapter 8 God's instructions to take Ai came again. This time, He told the Israelites to lie in ambush. They waited outside the city, and when the king and his people rode out to battle, the Israelites rose up from where they hid and defeated their enemy.

Pastor Goodman stayed on this series three or four weeks. Each week he repeated a lot of what he said the previous week, as often happens when anyone teaches a series to refresh the congregation's memory and to inform those who missed a week in the series. When he said he was going to preach on Joshua 8 for a third week, I took a deep sigh, and maybe even rolled my eyes, and prepared to utilize a lot of patience in listening to the repetition of what God had to say. I am so glad I listened with an open mind. It was no longer just a story to me as God spoke to me sometime after that sermon.

I was climbing into the shower when I believe I clearly heard God's voice.

"I want you to ambush your enemy and fight for the salvation of your family," came the command.

"Okay, Lord, how do I do that?"

"Using spiritual warfare."

"What spiritual warfare?"

"Through praise dancing."

"Okay. I will do that."

Then, I finished my shower and went to bed. By morning, I had decided the best thing to do (yes, I decided—I didn't even ask God) would be to join the dance ministry. I didn't know how to dance, really, so that seemed like the most logical place to start. I truly wanted to dance and worship God, and I was sure that making the sacrifice to dance in spite of my pain would lead to my healing, and maybe get my family saved. It was not an easy road to take, though.

One Sunday morning the pain struck in a way that made me even more determined to seek healing. I was dancing, enjoying my time in the Lord as I always did. That morning's dance leader, Michelle, was in the middle, and I was dancing on her left side. As I came out of a spin and stepped forward, my hip muscle tensed and my leg buckled. I almost fell, but I regained my composure and went on.

Michelle saw what happened and mouthed, "Are you okay?"

I shook my head "no," but I followed her lead until we were finished and she led us off the stage. Fortunately, this was an isolated incident. I never again felt like I would fall during worship, and the times my leg did nearly collapse were very seldom.

Our church soon had a week of nightly healing services. I was not anxious to ask for prayer, but I was still dancing every night, believing I was going to get a breakthrough, though I didn't know what it might be. My hip, or gluteus, pain was not the only pain I was experiencing at this time. I was still suffering migraines, as my healing from them did not come until many years later. I had also hurt my shoulder on the job, which I will talk more about later, but for now let me introduce you to just a little bit about it.

My left rotator cuff was hurt. The pain had increased to the point that by the time of those healing services, I could barely lift my arm. There were certain ways I could not lift it; my range of motion was very poor. This was the injury that was on my mind when I went to the altar for prayer one night. God had something else in mind.

As I sat and watched others getting prayer one night during this week of services, I noticed a recurring theme. The minister, whom I will call Jack because I don't remember his name, kept asking people about resentments they were harboring. I thought it curious that every person he asked confirmed Jack was correct, that they needed to forgive someone and release resentment or bitterness.

That night, as I went to prepare for bed, God's voice came to me, "You have resentment towards your daughter."

I immediately knew He was reminding me of the others I had seen getting prayer that night. I was also scared. I loved (and love) my Arienne. Resentment towards her had never knowingly entered my mind. I don't know what God meant by "resentment." Resentment for being born, for my being pregnant, or because my life's goals had been so affected by my pregnancy? I didn't know. I did know that sometimes Satan makes us feel condemned for things that aren't true when we see others receiving instruction in an area. It was on this premise that I based my prayer.

"Okay, God," I said as I brushed my hair in the mirror. "I don't know if that's You or not. I am not going to say it out loud because if it's not You, I don't want Satan to use it against me. If it is You, I ask that You confirm it through the man of God tomorrow night."

I went to bed not knowing what to expect, but hopeful nonetheless.

When Jack offered the altar call the next night, I went down for prayer. I wanted healing for my shoulder. He told us that the power to heal was not in him; it is in all of us as Believers. He wanted us to pray for ourselves. Jack first instructed us to put a hand on the part of our body that needed healing and to pray, and I did so. I put my right hand on my left shoulder and prayed. He then told us to move or do something we couldn't do before. He said that if we noticed something different, to let him know and he would come over and talk with us. I tested my range of motion by lifting and lowering my arm in various positions. My shoulder didn't hurt, so I motioned to Jack, who came right over.

"What's happening," he asked.

I told him, "I came down to get confirmation on something I believe God told me last night, but I prayed for my shoulder just now. I can move it in ways I couldn't before."

Jack then asked me about myself. "How many children do you have?"

"I have one daughter."

"How old is she?"

"She's seven."

I don't remember the other questions he asked, but it was the final thing Jack said to me that will always matter most.

"You need to come in and speak to your pastors. Pastor Goodman and his wife are great to talk to, and they'll be able to help you. And they will be glad to do it. Okay?"

"Yes," I nodded.

"You've got *good* pastors here," he repeated with emphasis.

I assured him I would come in and speak to the pastor and his wife as he instructed. The next day, I called to make an appointment with Pastor Goodman and his wife, Vicky.

I was in a lot of pain the day of my appointment. I gingerly walked in and sat across from Pastor Goodman with Vicky sitting next to me. I pushed the pain aside, stayed strong, and told them everything I could think of. In about 30 minutes, they knew my entire life's story.

How I had been sexually abused several times and raped twice. I told them of getting pregnant, and of meeting my husband a few months later. I told them how I came to be married to a nonbeliever even though I knew it was not God's will to do so. They heard how I believed God showed me I was resentful and bitter, and how Jack had in fact confirmed it, just as I had asked God to do. All of this had led to the moment that brought me to Pastor Goodman's office that day.

I finished by telling them a revelation I thought I had received about my husband. I was driving home one day when

I prayed, "God, why, after everything I've done to him, does Lee love me so much?" (I was referring to my behavior before we got married, which may someday be chronicled in another book.)

I felt God whisper, "Because he loves you as Christ loves the Church, like he's *supposed* to."

Pastor Goodman looked at me with compassion, "I agree with you," he said. "You have a husband who does love you as Christ loves the Church. I wish I could get some Christian men to love their wives that way."

"Thank you," I smiled. It was nice to finally feel as if someone could hear my story and not judge me for knowingly and intentionally marrying an unbeliever.

I continued on with my story. I told Pastor Goodman of the people who had told me I needed to confront my abusers—one abuser, in particular—if I wanted healing. I told him I didn't believe that was necessary.

He didn't hesitate to answer, "You know, Michelle, when it comes to confronting someone you have to consider whether it will be of benefit. If it isn't going to resolve anything, sometimes it is better to leave it alone."

"That's what I think," I told him. "If it isn't going to help, I don't see any reason in bringing it up."

I was relieved to have someone I respected so much agree with me. It wasn't that I refused to talk about it if the opportunity arose. I am never one to back down from voicing what I think I need to. I just understand that forgiveness is a choice, and you do it whether the offending party is sorry or not. You also forgive whether you ever confront the other person or not.

As I sat there talking to Pastor and Vicky Goodman, pouring out everything in me, I felt the pain in my hip leave. By the time our conversation ended, there was no pain in my hip at all.

I walked out of his office and never felt that pain again! My healing came as I let go of decades of accumulated resentment and bitterness. I learned firsthand what it means to prosper and be in good health as your soul prospers, and it was only the beginning of what God was going to teach me.

Interestingly, I still don't know what I was resentful of. I just know that a peaceful heart, one that lets go of the past and moves on in healthy and meaningful ways, results in a healthy body.

Surgery Heals

I am a firm believer that God uses doctors and surgery to heal. I know there are many who disagree with that statement. I have friends who say things like, "Doctors *practice* medicine. They don't know anything for sure." Or, "It is job security for doctors and pharmacists to keep you sick. They can treat you, but they can't cure you, nor do they want to." The funny thing is, these same friends will all go to the doctor and take the prescribed medicines because they do hold out some hope that doing so will help them.

While there may be some truth to their statements, I don't think they are completely accurate. I think good doctors are well-educated in their specific field, but they also know their limitations. I also believe most doctors and pharmacists are human beings who empathize with their patients and would like to see people well.

I am much more concerned with the pastors and preachers who act like we must live in "divine health" to truly experience the fullness of God. You know the ones I am talking about. Those pastors who never have a headache, who would have us believe that we are somehow lacking in faith if we get a cold or the flu.

I quit listening to all of them. I no longer give any attention to anyone who either discounts the real value of doctors or who thinks faith means never being sick. Yes, I believe God heals. Yes, I believe God's greatest desire is for us to live in perfect health, unaffected by the things we eat that should be good for us but sometimes aren't. But, I also know we are living in a fallen world.

From the moment sin entered the world, mankind has been prone to sickness and disease, and we will continue to be vulnerable until the world ends. That is just reality.

Because we are living in a fallen world, God gives doctors the wisdom and knowledge they need to help us live longer, healthier lives. Natural medicine, or naturopathy, is great, but even it can only do so much. Additionally, naturopathy often relies on New Age or Eastern medicine practices that Christians should not participate in. So, I go to the medical doctor when I need to, but I also do the things I can in my (often vain) attempts to avoid a trip to the doctor. Sometimes, though, I have no alternative *but* to see a doctor.

I really learned the benefit of modern medicine after my first two (out of seven) surgeries.

At this time, between 1997 and 2002, I worked off and on at a fire and smoke restoration company. When business slowed down, as often happens in service industries, the boss, Steve, kept us all busy by accepting a contract to clean up the new construction sites on Ft. Bragg, North Carolina. They were building new dental offices, and the construction sites had to be clean at all times, or the contractor risked being fined by the Army. Since the work crews could not stop to pick up waste and still get the job done in a timely manner, our company accepted the responsibility. We picked up and discarded all the debris you usually find on a construction site: electrical wires, empty spools, sheetrock, and more.

One day, as we worked on the new dental clinic, I was carrying a handful of sheetrock pieces to the dumpster. It had been a long day, though it was only the early afternoon. I could feel my muscles working extra hard to hold onto this particular load because it was heavier than most of the loads I had previously carried.

As I approached the dumpster, I felt a terrible pull in my left shoulder muscle, right at the very top of the joint. I have always heard that when you tear a rotator cuff—a group of tendons in the shoulder joint—you know it. I don't know if I tore the cuff that day, but I do know something happened to it. It wasn't painful enough to make me drop what was in my hands, and I was able to throw the sheetrock into the dumpster. So, I shook it off and kept on working.

Eventually, the pain in my shoulder grew worse. Over the next days or weeks, it got so bad I went to the doctor. He sent me to physical therapy. I wasn't too keen on the idea of therapy, given that my first experience went so poorly. I trusted the doctor, though, and hoped this time therapy would be different. It only ended the same way, though.

The therapist, Diane, seemed friendly. She talked to me a bit, and showed me the exercises she wanted me to do. We sat and talked at the end of my appointment. I mentioned I was seeing a chiropractor, and that was when it all went south.

"You can't see a chiropractor," Diane firmly stated.

"Oh, I don't see him for my shoulder. I see him for my back and hip," I kindly tried to reassure her. (Remember my hip pain had not been healed at this point.)

Her attitude went straight from firm to anger. "I know, but you can't be seen here if you are going to see a chiropractor."

"Not even for my back?"

"It doesn't matter," she nearly yelled. "You cannot be seen here in this office and see a chiropractor. If you are going to see a chiropractor, you can't come back."

I didn't go back. I have never gotten used to medical professionals yelling at me. I still didn't tolerate it well today, and I won't return to the office of someone who yells.

I did continue doing the exercises Diane gave me, though. I faithfully did them, too—until my shoulder quit hurting. Whenever my shoulder started hurting again, I practiced the exercises again, until it stopped hurting. Then, the cycle would start over again. I followed this pattern—pain, exercise, relief, no exercise, pain—for several years. Thirteen years, to be exact.

I had prayed for myself that night Jack was at our church, and it is true that after that prayer, my pain was relieved and I had my range of motion back. But, the pain returned sometime after that. I don't know when my shoulder started hurting again. I do know that 13 years after that night at the altar I once again couldn't lift my arm. I had lost all range of motion, and the pain was unbearable. The therapy exercises no longer helped. I could do them, but they no longer offered even the slightest pain relief. My family doctor prescribed Ultram, Ibuprofen, and Skelaxin. They helped me sleep when the pain kept me awake, but they didn't do much else. The doctor soon sent me to the orthopedist.

I was sure I wouldn't like Dr. Baines from the start. I sat in the waiting room for two hours before they called my name. I followed the nurse down a hallway that was eerily empty. There were a few pictures on the walls, but there was no other staff about. No one sat at the desk or walked between rooms. I sat and waited for another hour before Dr. Baines finally stepped in to see me. The exam did not take long. After seeing how much pain I was in, he prescribed Norco and ordered an MRI.

Let me take a moment to tell you about MRIs in case you have never had one. You lie on a narrow, concave bed. Most of the MRI beds remind me of a canoe, something on which you can lie down straight, but not lie flat, because of the way the body curves and pushes your shoulders and hips forward. The radiology tech will usually give you ear plugs and/or headphones to protect your ears from the loud buzzing noises the machine makes. The tech will ask if you are claustrophobic and will then give you a button to hold so you can push it, in case you have any issues while you are in the machine. With a few more simple instructions specific to your case, the tech pushes a button and the bed you are on slides into a very small tube. I am sure it is a large tube, but it seems so small. The top of it is only one to three inches from your face. The sides and bottom of the tube are so close that they are in contact with every available inch of your body. It is very nerve wracking, even to someone who does not have claustrophobia.

I have come to hate MRIs, or as Judy Garland's character said in *Meet Me in St. Louis*, I "loathe, despise, and abominate" them. You would think the more often I get them, the more I would get used to them. I guess, though, it is the anticipation of knowing what is going to happen that increases my anxiety, each MRI making me more nervous than the last. It is helpful when the radiology tech lets me pick the music she plays. I select a Christian station if I can, or I may opt for no music to be piped in, and instead quietly sing worship songs to myself. It is a great way to cope and helps me remember that Christ is in control of both the present situation and the results of the test.

So, I lay on the bed and the radiology tech gave me the usual instructions. She spoke with me throughout the test, letting me know the next segment of imaging would take 5 minutes, or 20 minutes, etc. The MRI was not nearly as dreadful as I had expected it to be. That is until it was time to get up. The awkward shape of the machine's bed made me very stiff, and it was impossible to move my shoulder at first. I had to very carefully turn myself over, one body part at a time, and sit up before I could rise off the bed, and even then the pain was excruciating. I can assure you I never wanted to go through that again!

I went back to Dr. Baines to find out what the radiologist's report said. My wait was not nearly as long this time, and I decided I would give him some mercy for making me wait so long at my previous visit. I really wanted to like Dr. Baines. I wanted him to find out what was wrong and fix it. I was tired of the pain and of trying to find a physical therapist I could connect with.

Dr. Baines gave me the bad news, "You have bone spurs on your left shoulder."

"Okay," I said, trying to remember if I had ever heard of bone spurs. I hadn't.

"You seem to have a small tear in your rotator cuff, too."

"Oh," came my more frightened response. Now, *that* I had heard of! "That's a six-week recovery period, right?"

"Yes," Dr. Baines confirmed. "But, it could be too small to repair. I just won't know how large it is until I get in there to remove the bone spurs. If the tear in the rotator cuff is large enough to repair, then I will. If it's too small, though, I will leave it alone."

This puzzled me. Why *not* fix it while you are in there? I didn't really care about the details, though, the hows and whys of what makes a rotator cuff repairable and what doesn't. I just wanted use of my arm again.

I went to the scheduling desk and we scheduled the surgery for November 3, 2010. My first surgery of six would be 30 days prior, October 3, on my left thumb. I will cover more about my thumbs and hands in another chapter. But, I will tell you that both surgeries were done, within one month of each other, both on the left side…and I am left handed. Fortunately, I am rather ambidextrous, and I easily learned to do many more things with my right hand during this time.

Dr. Baines performed the surgery on my left shoulder. I was attending post-operative physical therapy, and I seemed to be healing as well as a body should. Until one night as I got in the tub. I put my hands in the water behind me to help myself sink lower. I felt my left shoulder tear—again. And it *hurt!* I was so scared about what I might have done to it, I ended my bath immediately and went to bed to rest my shoulder.

When I saw Dr. Baines again, I told him I had re-injured my shoulder. He ordered another MRI. According to the radiologist's report, I had in fact torn the rotator cuff worse than it was prior to the surgery, but not bad enough for Dr. Baines to repeat the surgery and fix it. Instead, he gave me a cortisone shot. It hurt so badly I nearly came up off the table and reached out as if I thought I might take the needle from him. I made a promise to myself then that I would never let anyone give me another cortisone shot. I broke that promise, of course, but I have learned so much through all these different journeys that I am certain no one will ever give me that shot again. I can't even recommend them to other people because of my own experiences.

Finally, though, I began to heal. I had two six-week prescriptions for therapy, and it took about a year before full range of motion returned to my shoulder. But, in the years since my full recovery—nine as of this writing—my left shoulder has not given me another moment's trouble.

I rejoice that God uses skilled doctors to bring healing. No Christian should ever feel unworthy or like they don't have enough faith just because they are not healed miraculously. Pray for a miracle, yes, but also utilize the doctors who have the wisdom and knowledge to treat our bodies with science and medicine.

Two Thumb Issues, Two Solutions

In addition to the long-sought-after healing for migraines and my hip, I have experienced at least one healing that was quick and without any drama. It didn't take years of doctors and research, only a moment or two.

In 2006, while we still lived in North Carolina, I went through a few months of pain and swelling in the thumb area of both of my palms. There was no explanation, no injury, that could help the doctor reach a reasonable diagnosis.

It was a great nuisance. The swelling would come and go, but it never seemed too bad. I could keep the pain to a minimum by wearing bowler's positioners, something rigid that prevented awkward twists in my wrists. Of course wearing them caused people to ask if I had carpal tunnel syndrome, so I didn't like wearing the positioners more than what was needed to make it through a day without pain. I didn't need the doubt and fear too many negative comments on my wrists might bring.

I went to the doctor, who referred me to a hand specialist. The specialist hooked my hands up to this machine with probes or "needles" that measured my tendons' thickness as they passed through my wrist bones.

The test was negative. I did not have carpal tunnel.

Even after the desirable results of the carpal tunnel test, my thumbs went through about a week of swelling. Nothing would effectively relieve my discomfort or diminish the swelling.

As I walked up to the front porch of our home one hot, summer day, I tripped. Whether it was over my own feet or the concrete sidewalk, I don't know. I fell forward, and my face rapidly proceeded toward the brick steps. I threw my hands straight out in front of me, and I landed squarely on the areas of my thumbs that had been swollen for the previous few months.

Now, if you know anything about falling you know you are supposed to make every effort *not* to put your hands out to catch yourself. Doing so can easily fracture your hands and wrists. A few years later I would learn that lesson from experience.

Nonetheless, after this first fall, I did catch myself with my hands. Then I stood up, massaged both of my palms, and prayed. "Lord, I don't know what is going on with my hands, but You do. I pray that, whatever is wrong with them, this fall was just what I needed to knock everything back into place."

In that moment, my thumbs were healed, and I never again had problems with their randomly swelling and hurting.

The next time I fell face-first, I did not fair quite as well. In January 2010 I was putting the trash out on the curb so it could be picked up the next morning. We lived in downtown Mount Holly, New Jersey, in a third-floor walk-up. The curb where our trash was picked up was only a sidewalk's width, about 24 inches, away from our building's front door. Like every other January in New Jersey, it was very cold, and I really did not want to step fully outside. Instead, I stood in the doorway, in about the middle of the sidewalk. I held the door open with one hand, while I threw my trash bag just a few inches away onto the pile of bags already on the street with my other hand.

This was a big mistake. As my arm swung the bag forward, the rest of my body tried to go with it. I stumbled on the welcome mat, and proceeded to topple forward just as I had four years prior in North Carolina. As with that first fall, I stuck my hands out in front of me. This time, though, it led to a serious injury.

The palms of my hands landed on one of the metal waste baskets that lined our street. I landed in a way that caused my thumb to hyperextend, and I knew immediately I had sprained it. I got Arienne to ride to the hospital with me. She didn't have her license yet, so she couldn't drive me, but I liked the comfort of having her there.

I made us both nervous driving those country roads to the hospital in Browns Mills with my right hand doing the steering. Since I was both left handed and in extreme pain, suddenly switching steering hands was probably not advisable. But, we made it, and the x-ray thankfully showed nothing was seriously wrong; nothing was broken.

Unfortunately, no matter what the x-ray showed, my thumb did not heal. In August it was still swollen and often in pain. I went to the base doctor and requested a referral to the hand surgeon.

Dr. Thompson was quite upset that the electronic copy of the x-rays I brought with me would not open on his computer. He could not see what was going on inside of my hand.

He put me through a few range of motion tests.

"Does this hurt?"

"Yes."

Does that hurt?

"No."

"Okay. You have trigger thumb."

"Okay."

"There are two options. I can give you a cortisone shot right there, in that tendon," he said as he held my hand, palm up, and showed me where the shot would go at the base of my thumb. "Or, we can perform what is called 'trigger finger' surgery. I would make a small incision right there in the line at the bottom of your thumb so it minimizes scarring. I would cut the tendon, and that would be it."

"Oh." Since this would be my first surgery, ever, I was a little apprehensive, and my face and voice showed it.

"Would you like to try a cortisone shot first?"

"Sure. That's fine."

I had not received a cortisone shot up to this point, so I knew very little about them. I found out later that the reason you can only have a certain number of cortisone shots to the same area within a specific period of time is that too much cortisone to an area actually deteriorates the bone—the opposite of what you want to do to someone who has bone issues.

Looking back, I remember receiving the shot, though I don't remember any pain associated with it. I also remember that it didn't work. What I don't remember, however, is the pain. Future cortisone shots would hurt so badly I would want to jump off the table, but I hardly felt a thing when Dr. Thompson administered the shot.

"Now," he explained when he had finished the injection, "It could be up to two days before you feel any relief, and then it should last about two weeks."

"Okay."

"Let's follow-up in two weeks so you can tell me how you're feeling. We can decide then if you will need surgery or not."

"I will, Dr. Thompson. Thank you."

The follow-up appointment was just as simple as the first.

"How did you react to the shot, Michelle? Are you feeling any better?"

"Well, it didn't take two days for the pain to stop. It stopped almost immediately."

"That's good news."

"Yeah, except that after those two days it was as if I never had the shot in the first place. It hurts as badly now as it ever did."

Dr. Thompson had options to offer. "Do you want to try another shot, or go ahead with surgery? Two shots are all I can give you. If the second one doesn't work, you are going to have to have the surgery anyway."

"I think I will just go ahead with the surgery, then."

He smiled, "That's a good idea. Let's get it scheduled."

The surgery was performed October 3, 2010. My physical therapy was very minimal. They gave me nothing more than stretching exercises. I was grateful for them, and how they restored my thumbs' range of motion, but the exercises were so minimal that they didn't help me get any strength back in my thumb. The swelling was gone, and the pain had been relieved, but I needed something more than just stretches. So, when I started seeing a therapist after the surgery on my left shoulder, I told him of the difficulty I was having with my thumb. He gave me some exercises to do, using a rubber band in the same way you would use a Thera-band for exercising larger parts of the body.

It pleases me to tell you that after learning those exercises, my thumb has not given me any more problems. It healed well, and has full strength and flexibility.

I am grateful for the many opportunities I have had to be healed. I wish I knew why God has sometimes healed me instantly or miraculously, while allowing me to go through surgeries other times. I do know that no matter what path of healing you seek, God is right there. He will work it all out to His glory and to your good, if you will trust Him and seek Him in all things.

The Spark of Hope
That Fizzled Out

In 2008, about a year or so after we moved to New Jersey, I started an intense boot camp-style fitness program. I soon noticed a sharp pain in my feet during certain exercises.

The pain first hit me during jumping jacks, which are mostly done on the balls of the feet. The pain's intensity was amplified by the jumping jacks if we did any running or other exercises first. I tried to "baby" my feet as much as possible, but the nature of the boot camp was such that we were expected to keep pace with our "teammates."

One day, the pain was so bad I just couldn't run. Running, you may not know (I didn't until this class), is done on the balls of the feet. You do not land on your whole foot or on your heel like you do in jogging or speed walking because that slows you down. You run on your "tiptoes" to run faster.

"What's wrong, Michelle," Terry asked as he ran alongside me one day after the pain and its frequency had increased to the point of making boot camp unbearable.

Am I limping? Maybe he just noticed I was walking instead of running.

"My feet hurt," I replied.

"We just need to get some strength in them. That's all."

"Yeah," I shrugged my shoulders doubtfully.

I tried to believe him. After all, I knew it couldn't hurt to strengthen my feet, and I was feeling more energetic after working out every morning. I didn't want to quit boot camp because I was sure exercise would help with my general fatigue. Not to mention it would help me lose the weight I needed.

But, the pain was not subsiding. Pretty soon it went from hurting during exercise to hurting all the time. I could just flex my foot or flick my ankle, and an unbelievably sharp pain would shoot through the arch of my foot. In short order, my feet hurt all the time. They didn't need any stimulation. They just hurt, and once they hurt, there was nothing I could do about it. I could only rest until the pain dissipated on its own.

I went to the doctor. He sent me to a podiatrist, Dr. Cobb.

Dr. Cobb's office staff were friendly. I liked them right away. It wasn't so with Dr. Cobb. I remember looking at him and thinking, *He doesn't look like a doctor. He looks like he should be on the cover of* GQ. It was more than just his thick, dark, wavy hair. No, there was something in his attitude that made me wonder if he was "in it for the money." I had never thought that about a doctor until that moment. I had always had much love and respect for doctors.

Dr. Cobb came in and examined my feet.

"Here's what I would like to do, Michelle. I would like to give you custom orthotics, shoe inserts."

"Okay. Sure."

"The military won't pay for them, though. They only pay for custom inserts for active duty members, not their dependents."

"Oh. How much are they?"

He quoted the price. I don't remember what he said, but it was a few hundred dollars. I think it was around $400.

"Unfortunately, you have a birth defect. There's nothing, really, that can be done about that."

"Oh," was the only confused response I could manage. On the one hand I thought, *You're the doctor. I need to trust you. On the other hand*, I thought, *if that's true, why has it gone undetected before now?*

"Well, if they will help. Sure. I will get the inserts."

Dr. Cobb put plaster on my feet and made molds of them. The shoe inserts would be made from these molds, and his office would contact me and let me know when they were ready.

When I returned to Dr. Cobb's office for what I had hoped would be my relief, I was immediately disappointed.

The shoe inserts he gave me were foam. Tiny, mish-mashed particles of foam pressed together like a jigsaw puzzle. They looked like the foam padding you lay under carpet. It was no surprise to me when these supposed arch "supports" were just as weak as the carpet foam they resembled. I did try to wear them a few days, including to boot camp. When they didn't help, I tossed them in the closet and never used them again.

Dr. Cobb did not do much for the reputation of doctors in general, but he did even less for my opinion of podiatrists. The worthless inserts had cost us hundreds of dollars, and I was sure they were my only hope, because, as he said, I had a birth defect that couldn't be helped, right?

So, I quit going to the doctor for my foot pain. For a while, I was able to simply abstain from most activities that aggravated the pain. I quit boot camp and rested a lot at home. For the most part, the pain subsided, but the relief didn't last long, and when the pain came back it was worse than before.

My regular doctor at the base was not available when I decided to try seeking treatment again. Since he was deployed, I had to see the lieutenant filling in for him. The lieutenant was rude and blamed me for all of my foot pain.

"You have plantar fasciitis," the lieutenant informed me.

"Okay," I said with a questioning look. I knew very little about the ailment, but I knew my dad had been diagnosed with it. All I could think was, *Aren't I a little young for that?*

"You need to lose weight," he scolded.

"I can't exercise, though. My feet hurt too badly."

"Well, until you lose weight they are going to hurt. What kind of shoes do you wear at home?"

"I don't wear shoes in the house. I go barefoot."

The lieutenant shot back, "You have to wear shoes, even inside. Plantar fasciitis is caused by fallen arches. Shoes are made today in a way that our feet become dependent on them. You can't go without them."

His humiliating and condescending attitude didn't stop there.

"Do you wear high heels," he asked.

"Oh, once in a while, but not much." A chiropractor had once warned me not to wear them more than once a week, and I did my best to comply, saving them for church and special occasions.

"Uh huh," he said, "that's why your toes are like that."

The lieutenant was referring to the large "hump" my pinky toes have. They are large and swollen compared to my other toes, and have always reminded me of a back crippled by osteoporosis. They have been that way since I was a child. I let him know that.

"Oh, they have been like that forever," I informed him, and I meant it quite literally.

He looked at me and said, "Yeah," with an attitude and a look that said, "I know…since you first started wearing heels."

I knew he was a lost cause and wouldn't listen, so I didn't bother trying to convince him my toes had truly been shaped like that all my life. I went home with the information the lieutenant had given me. I did the exercises and stretches detailed on the printouts he sent home with me, but they didn't help. The pain got worse. I once again gave up seeking help for a little while. When I finally did ask to see a podiatrist again, my search became the longest and most difficult period of my life.

My husband had begun to see a podiatrist for his own foot problems. His issues were much worse than mine, with deformed bone in each foot, which had to be removed. But, he liked his doctor, Dr. Hopewell. If a man who never goes to the doctor, and who can't stand strangers touching him, tells you he likes a particular doctor, you can be sure the doctor is probably a good one. I returned to the base, where my doctor was back from deployment, and requested to be sent to Dr. Hopewell. I was glad I did, but my joy was short-lived.

Dr. Hopewell assured me that everything both Dr. Cobb and the lieutenant had told me was wrong. He said I did not have a birth defect, and that neither my weight nor my desire to go barefoot had any bearing on my plantar fascia pain. Yes! I felt totally affirmed and even a little vindicated in my disbelief towards the other two doctors.

As with all doctors, Dr. Hopewell started me on the conservative first step of choice. He instructed me to get the shoe inserts he recommended. All doctors have a different brand and style of shoe inserts they prefer. I eventually saw seven doctors total about my feet, and no two of them agreed on which inserts were best. He also prescribed physical therapy, and I was having some success. I looked forward to seeing Dr. Hopewell through my entire healing process, but he soon fell ill, and got so sick that he ended up selling his practice.

At first I saw one of Dr. Hopewell's substitutes who was kind enough to temporarily accept his patients. By this time, the pain in my feet was something more than just the plantar fasciitis. I had developed a pain between my toes that caused unbearable pain in my second and third toes with every step I took. Dr. Jackson diagnosed me with a pinched nerve in my toes on both feet. That was the diagnosis I expected, but, he wanted to operate and insert a plastic v-shaped stint between my toes to separate them. I didn't feel right about his prognosis. I just needed time to think about it, so I decided I wouldn't go back until I had decided whether I would go forward with the surgery.

Although I was at a complete loss as to what to do about my plantar fasciitis, and relief was still many years ahead of me, I soon had the answer to my "pinched nerve" problem. During my quiet time with God, I pondered my most recent diagnosis and my repulsion at the thought of that stint being implanted into my foot. I believe the Holy Spirit gave me the answer.

I began to think of all the times my foot bones are "squished" together. I thought of the shoes I wore. Yes, I wore heels, but not that often, and since the pain was persistent, I figured it had to be something I did more frequently. I thought of the non-heels I wore. My tennis shoes, my flats. Some of the doctors I had already seen recommended shoes with a lot of wiggle room in the toes, or the toe box, as it is officially called. Assuming that tight shoes put too much pressure on my toes, doctors thought I needed room to flex my toes more easily.

However, I realized that tighter shoes, in spite of conventional wisdom, actually relieved the pain more than shoes that were loose in the toes. Tighter shoes held my toes still instead of letting them slide and flop around like they did in looser shoes, or like they did when I was barefoot. But, I knew that how my shoes fit was probably only a contributing factor, and not the final answer.

I thought of all the times I sat with my legs crossed "Indian style." Yes, surely sitting with the weight of my leg resting firmly on my foot on a regular basis did not help. I quit sitting that way, and the pain got better, but did not stop. There was still more to what I was doing to cause this pinched nerve issue. I saw a vision of myself sleeping. I realized that, at that time, I slept with my legs and feet wrapped around and tucked under my husband's leg. I considered for a moment that just maybe my pinched nerve was caused by my sleeping habits. I began to consciously avoid sleeping with my legs wrapped around my husband. I simply lay next to him instead. After just a few nights, the pain was gone!

Well, that was one foot pain resolved, but not all of them. I still had the plantar fasciitis to deal with. The physical therapist I was seeing for some new issues that had developed (things I will tell you of later) suggested I see the sports medicine doctor in her building. I had seen him before, so I was familiar with him. I call him Dr. Malkovich because I think he so closely resembled John Malkovich.

Dr. Malkovich had recently become certified in a method called Tenex, a process developed by the Mayo Clinic. It is a method used to respire (suck) the scarred tissue out of the body at the site of certain ailments. Besides treating plantar fasciitis, the non-surgical procedure can help patients with tennis elbow, jumper's knee, and Achilles' tendonitis. Dr. Malkovich had performed the procedure on other patients who had experienced some success, so I was very hopeful I would, too.

The procedure was performed on each foot separately. Since this was a non-surgical procedure, I would be awake the entire time. When he did the first foot, Dr. Malkovich only gave me a local anesthetic, assuring me that was all I needed. I was in a lot of pain through the entire procedure. It is hard to sit still when you are in constant pain, but jerking or moving increases the risks of the procedure. The recovery went well, though, and when the second foot was to be taken care of, Dr. Malkovich admitted he would have to do something more to stave off the pain. He agreed to numbing my foot more effectively with a nerve blocker.

The second procedure went a lot more smoothly, with my foot fully numb from the shot he gave me. As Dr. Malkovich made the incision and inserted and then maneuvered the suction wand, I didn't feel a thing. When he admitted that he would have to use a nerve blocker on future patients, I wondered how his past patients had faired with only the local anesthetic he had administered during my first procedure. I hoped they had not suffered as much as I had.

With both procedures completed, I recovered quickly, and hoped that I could avoid surgery. That was supposed to be one of the greatest benefits of Tenex, not having to go through either an open or arthroscopic surgery.

In only a couple of years, I would soon find that I was not so lucky as to avoid surgery. I had once been so hopeful that a simple aspiration technique would be a permanent solution. It was not. Help would eventually come, but not until after I saw a few more doctors.

The Podiatrists
with No Heart

When we moved from New Jersey to Georgia, I naturally had to find all new doctors. I knew I would eventually need an orthopedist, but I thought I needed a good podiatrist first.

I moved to Georgia ahead of Lee. He had another year in the Air Force before he could take leave and prepare for retirement. I came early so that I could make sure the house was in order and determine who would be in what bedrooms. My mother-in-law, Tommie; Arienne; and my granddaughter, Ada, were already in the home Lee and I planned to move into, so there was much to prepare. I also wanted a job in our new location. I needed to start before Lee retired. With both of us working, we could get more savings together in case Lee did not find a job immediately after retirement.

Soon, Arienne and I had a bit of a falling out. She moved to Acworth, about an hour's drive from our house. I couldn't stand the thought of being without my precious Ada. Every weekend, I drove to Acworth and picked her up. She stayed with her Granny, as all the grandchildren call Tommie, and me from Friday to Sunday, when I would drive her home.

My feet had already started hurting again by this point, and the four-way drive every weekend quickly proved to be overwhelming. I attributed it to the stop and go traffic that Atlanta and the metro area are so famous for. Since I didn't think it was anything more than the drive, I didn't think too much of it at first. But, as the pain increased I decided to seek treatment once again.

My doctor issued a referral to Dr. Frost, a very nice podiatrist who seemed eager to help me. The first time I saw Dr. Frost, she did not jump to prescribing a specific orthotic. Nor did she try to get me to accept a cortisone shot. Instead, she made some cushions of her own.

"I am not going to give you a cortisone shot," Dr. Frost said.

"Good. I don't think they are very helpful, and they hurt so badly," I was relieved.

"I just don't think they would do much good until you get some of this inflammation down. When you have been in pain as long as you have, they don't tend to help."

"Oh, okay," I said as I thought, *I don't really care what the reason is. I'm just glad I don't need one.*

"I am going to make you something here, though," she said as she grabbed her scissors and some tape.

I was intrigued as I watched Dr. Frost work. First, she cut a length of strong, wide medical tape similar in color to an Ace bandage. She formed the tape into a cylindrical shape, with the adhesive on the outside. Then, she took a piece of foam she had cut to the shape of my right foot and placed it on the tape. Finally, she wrapped the first tape cylinder with a second piece of the same tape, but with the adhesive on the inside. She drew an R and an arrow on the top of the "homemade" arch support so I would know which foot it should be worn on and in what direction. She repeated the same process to make an arch support for the left foot.

"You have to wear these every day, unless you are sleeping."

"Sure, I can do that," I shrugged.

I left her office a little hopeful since her homemade arch cushions seemed to relieve the pain almost immediately. When I went back to Dr. Frost, I was happy to report that the arch supports seemed to help a lot. But, by the third visit the arch supports were no longer of benefit. She had still more non-surgical solutions in mind.

Dr. Frost told me, "I am going to give you plantar fasciitis boots to sleep in."

"Okay. Does my insurance pay for them?"

"I don't know for sure, but we will bill the insurance company first, and then whatever they don't cover we will bill you for the difference."

"Of course. That's fine."

The boots were huge! I had never seen such devices, but since the arch supports Dr. Frost had made helped so much (however temporarily), I decided to trust her and give them a try. She made me fresh arch supports with tape and foam and sent me on my way, until the next follow-up appointment.

Those sleeping boots were the worst "remedy" I would experience in all of my plantar fasciitis journey. The boots looked similar to walking casts—the firm but removable cast that doctors often prescribe for minor fractures and other ailments of the foot. They were much larger than walking casts, though. More like space boots, it seemed to me. The difference was that the sleeping boots had flat bottoms, instead of a curved bottom like casts have. In fact, the sleeping boots come with explicit instructions not to walk in them (not that you *can* walk when you have both of them on). I tried it once, and nearly fell on my face.

I knew from the first night that the sleeping boots would not last long. Still, I tried to give them a chance to work. After a couple of weeks, I gave up. The boots were clunky enough when worn individually. Wearing two at the same time was a literal nightmare. I couldn't turn over in bed with both of them on, so I was constantly waking up just to make sure my feet turned over with the rest of my body. Such repeated interruptions made a good night's sleep impossible. In addition, I quickly realized that my feet worked against the boots. The boots are supposed to keep your foot at a 90-degree angle so that the calf muscles and Achilles' tendons stay stretched enough to be relaxed through the night, and thus prevent the patient from waking in pain in the morning. My feet, though, pointed down against the sole of the boots and stayed tense all night, thus defeating the purpose of the boots. To make matters even worse, I often wouldn't keep them on all night. Many mornings I awakened to find the boots had been removed and laid on the floor or lost in the covers. I had no idea how they had been removed and could only deduce they had been so uncomfortable that I took them off in my sleep.

I reported all of this to Dr. Frost. Her answer was to prescribe physical therapy.

Naturally, by this time I was familiar with physical therapy and the exercises I would have to do. But, also by this time, I was familiar enough with both therapy and my body to have very little confidence in the relief she promised would come. I went to a few therapy sessions and reported the results back to Dr. Frost.

"Well, the therapy doesn't seem to be helping, but maybe it will."

She again made the custom medical tape arch supports. As her head was down, looking at my feet I said, "You know, you might have to just do the surgery."

Without looking up at me, she shook her head with a sly smile and said, "Noooo, you don't qualify for surgery. No, no, no."

"Oh."

I didn't understand why she would have that reaction, but it wasn't her answer that put me off as much as her lack of communication skills and her attitude. It was like she was laughing at me. Her "no, no, no" had all the air of "tsk, tsk, tsk," and the slight laugh in her voice and the teasing smile on her face told me she was not taking me seriously at all.

I left her office unsure of whether I would ever return. But, I did still have another appointment with my physical therapist. They helped me make the final decision.

On my next visit to physical therapy, the therapist who had initially assessed my condition was not in. It gave me a chance to talk openly with the ones who were there. I recounted to them the years-long struggle I had already been through to find relief for my foot pain.

"I just don't think therapy is going to do much good," I admitted.

One of the therapists agreed, "You are right. After so many years, it is likely that surgery may *be* your best option."

"I know, but when I mentioned the possibility of surgery to Dr. Frost she laughed me off. She couldn't even look at me as she shook her head and said with a smile that I didn't even qualify for the surgery."

"Why would she say that?" He continued, "It is good to have a doctor who doesn't want to jump right into surgery, but you need one who is willing to do it if that is what you need."

"Thank you! I agree."

Another therapist joined the conversation. "Really? I have a patient who is about your age who just had the same surgery."

"You do? Can you give me the doctor's name?"

As she opened a file, she said, "That's just what I'm doing. Let me see if I can get his name for you. Yep. It's right here."

"Oh, thank you! I will call him. Where is his office?"

She explained to me where it was, and I recognized it immediately from her description. In fact, it is hard not to know where this particular doctor is. His office is at a major intersection of two local highways.

"Thank you so much. This is wonderful. I hope he will help."

"I think he will," she said. "Our other patient really seems to like him, and he is a good doctor."

I headed home finally hopeful again. I had the name of a doctor who might be willing to help, and I had the support of physical therapists who agreed surgery might be my best option.

The doctor the therapist recommended was on my way home, so I decided to stop in and see if he could help me. I figured if they could, I would make an appointment immediately. If he couldn't, at least I wouldn't have to wait any longer to find out. The receptionist was very friendly.

"May I help you," she asked as she slid the privacy glass open.

"Hi, I got your name from my physical therapist. I was wondering if you accept Tricare Prime."

"We don't accept Tricare Prime as a primary insurance. It has to be a secondary insurance only."

"Oh, no, that won't help me. Let me ask you this. Do you have another doctor you recommend who does take Tricare?"

"Yes, we normally refer to Dr. Cross."

She wrote Dr. Cross's name and number on a sticky note and handed it to me. I thanked her and left. From my regular doctor, I got the referral needed to see Dr. Cross and made the appointment.

Thankfully, he had an immediate opening. By this time the pain had increased to a level I didn't even know existed. I was fantasizing all kinds of strange things.

At one point, I had pondered the idea of never walking again. I thought life consigned to a wheelchair couldn't be that bad, and that maybe I could just get used to staying off my feet forever. I was in too much pain to concern myself with how impractical this would be, considering I would have to get around to go to the bathroom or get in and out of bed. Some days the pain was so unbearable I fantasized cutting my feet off.

If I got my feet caught in a bear trap, I reasoned, *I would have to cut my feet off, and then it wouldn't seem like I was doing it just because the pain had driven me to insanity.*

But, when you are in as much pain as I was, insanity comes easily.

I told Dr. Cross of the years of trouble I had experienced with my feet.

"It was so bad one day, that I couldn't even stand up from sitting on the couch. Every time I bent my *knee* to stand up, my *foot* hurt so badly I couldn't move. I had to get down on the floor and crawl to the TV."

"Don't do that," he scolded a little stronger than a doctor ever should.

I was shocked, as our conversation had been pretty calm until this point.

"I had to," I winced, "it hurt too bad to walk. I couldn't even stand up." I am sure I was near the point of tears.

"I know," said Dr. Cross, "but if you don't get up and walk on it anyway, you are only going to make it worse."

The rest of the visit was pretty typical, compared to all my other doctors.

As I expected by now, Dr. Cross's first prescription was for me to buy a specific orthotic, or shoe insert. I was skeptical, but I obeyed his request, knowing that refusal would only make him less willing to help me. He had further instructions for me, though.

"I want you to walk like this," he said as he demonstrated placing the heel down on the ground and rolling the foot through to complete the step.

"Okay. I can do that. That's how we marched in band."

I was trying to compare his instructions to something I could relate to so I could be sure I was doing it right. But Dr. Cross was just being disagreeable that day, and wouldn't confirm anything I said.

"No, not like band. I want you to do it like this."

"Oh. Okay." No matter what he said, it looked the same as marching band to me, but I wasn't going to argue.

"I also want you to stretch twenty times like this five times a day." He showed me how to plant my heel next to a wall and place the rest of my foot on the wall to stretch the back of my calf and the Achilles' tendon.

"Okay. Sure." I said, knowing the exercise well after of all the other podiatrists and therapists I had already seen.

"Come back and see me in three months."

I did just as Dr. Cross said. I stretched as often as he told me, and I walked the way he showed me. I ordered the shoe inserts he recommended. Nothing helped. The pain did not get any better, and by the time I saw Dr. Cross again, *I* was a little cross!

"How have you been, Michelle?" he asked at my second appointment.

"It hasn't gotten any better, Dr. Cross. My ankles and feet are swollen all the time, and I have to take Norco just to make it through the day."

"You just have to keep stretching it and walking the way I showed you. Did you get the inserts I prescribed?"

"Yes, but none of it is working. I have been dealing with this so long. Do you see why I want to seek a *permanent* solution?" I was referring to surgery, of course, and he got the hint.

"I know you do," he started agreeably enough, "but if you don't get some flexibility in that ankle, surgery is not going to do you any good." That was the end of his agreeableness.

He continued, "Now, I want you to continue the stretches and come back and see me again in three more months."

I was a little reluctant to agree to waiting another three months, but I was hopeful about the fact that Dr. Cross at least seemed to believe surgery was a viable option for my plantar fasciitis. If I had known what he would say at the next three-month appointment, I would not have returned to his office that one last time.

My next and final appointment went the same way as all my previous appointments with Dr. Cross. He asked how I was, we talked a bit about my condition, and he told me to go home and stretch every day for three more months.

I was so despondent that he did not truly give me any hope for healing that I never returned. I just couldn't see him again. I was sure someone would eventually help me. I had no idea who or when, but I was done hoping it would be Dr. Cross.

The Orthopedist
from Heaven

I generally balk at the idea of giving heavenly attributes to human beings. But, if any doctor could be honored enough to be called my angel, it would be Dr. Davis. Unfortunately, it would be a while before I found him.

Shortly after the surgery on my left shoulder was completed and I finished my physical therapy, I started experiencing some pain in my right shoulder. I went to a doctor who prescribed physical therapy. I had already been through therapy, when I had the left shoulder operated on. My therapists believed in being symmetrical. So, when they worked my left shoulder, they also worked the right. But, since surgery is something we all should avoid if possible, I agreed to go specifically for the right shoulder. Plus, I knew it was a first step, that if I wanted something more done I would have to go through the nonsurgical processes first.

My right shoulder issues had everyone stumped, including my therapist. She and my doctor agreed that my right shoulder had an impingement, meaning something limited my range of motion, but nothing showed on the MRI. There were no visible bone spurs, like there had been on the left shoulder. All indications were that physical therapy would strengthen my shoulder and give me the pain relief I needed. My new physical therapist was trained in a technique called Active Release Therapy (A.R.T.). She would use her thumb to put pressure on specific points in my shoulder tendons and joint while simultaneously moving my shoulder through a range of motions. The technique worked really well. I always felt better after a session, and I was hopeful that the therapy was going to heal my shoulder.

By the time three years had passed, my right shoulder very clearly showed signs of having the same bone spurs my left shoulder had. I had lost all range of motion and could not lift my arm above waist-high. If I slept on my right side, I could not move my right arm at all the next morning. Getting dressed was about the most I could do. Since there is a muscle that runs along the back, connecting one shoulder to the other, I even had to be careful how high I lifted my left arm. Hanging clothes, for instance, with my left hand, sent me reeling from the pain it triggered in my right shoulder. I was in agony.

I had moved to Georgia by the time the pain in my right shoulder had reached its most debilitating point, and though I had family, I didn't have my husband who was still in New Jersey. It was not easy to once again experience that kind of pain without him. I had already gone through having my gall bladder removed without him in December 2013. I really did not want to face another surgery "alone."

By the summer of 2014, I had to start finding help for the right shoulder, though, and so I started in the usual place. I researched doctors who were in my insurance provider's network. I looked at their websites and decided the one I thought would be best. I went to my doctor and asked for the required referral.

I didn't know I had chosen one of the worst doctors imaginable. I don't even know if I want to give him a name, my experience was so miserable. He was young and still "by the book," and I will admit the pain had given me a bit of an attitude. I went into his office knowing what I wanted, and fully expecting him to agree. Having three surgeries between October 2010 and December 2013, one of which was preceded by the exact symptoms I was currently having, gave me a bit of arrogant assurance in knowing what I needed.

This doctor did not agree. His computer would not access the MRI files I took with me, so he ordered his own x-rays be done on the spot. While the radiology technicians were processing the images, they showed me to an exam room where I waited briefly for the doctor. When he entered the room, he came in like a whirlwind. A doctor who comes in that fast tends to move patients out that fast, and even worse, they usually don't listen to me. That's always bad, not listening to me, whether you are a doctor or not. I can still get pretty childish about it. Interacting with this doctor was no exception.

The doctor took me through the usual steps to check my range of motion. He had me lift my arm, straight out, to shoulder level. He pressed down to test my strength. He did the same thing with my arm straight out to my right, pressing down to test it. Then, he had me bend my elbows in front of me and plant them at my waist. I grabbed his hands with each of mine and pulled them towards me. I took the same position and he pulled my hands toward him. None of this hurt immediately, but it was very clear I had no strength at all.

The doctor was firm, "I am going to prescribe physical therapy."

"Ok. What about surgery?"

"According to what I see on the x-ray, and given your age, I can't do the surgery."

"But, it feels the same as when I had the surgery on my left shoulder, and I can't function. It really is affecting my quality of life."

That phrase "quality of life" seemed to be a trigger for him. It is a phrase doctors often use when they know they have to justify surgery and procedures to insurance companies, but it isn't one they expect patients to know well. But, those same doctors don't like it when a patient seems so arrogant as to use it when requesting help from the doctor.

"Again," he repeated obviously on the verge of anger, "according to what I see on the x-ray, and given your age, surgery really is not recommended. Now, I am going to prescribe physical therapy, and you can come back and see me in four to six weeks."

I resigned. "Okay…" was all I could muster. Urging him to see my point of view was futile.

The doctor moved toward the door, and as he started to open it, the pain from the strength and motion tests he put me through hit me all at once. The pain struck me like a lightning bolt, and I held nothing back. In the middle of his telling me to go to physical therapy for a third time, I screamed from the pain.

Did my pain phase him? No. I do realize the look on my face was questioning, searching his to see if my obvious pain was having an effect on him. I knew, even in the throes of pain, that such a look could make me seem manipulative, but I really wasn't trying to be. It truly hurt just as badly as I let on.

The doctor opened the door and told me he would see me in a month or so. I left the exam room, thinking he probably would not. His front desk confirmed what I already knew.

The receptionist handed me the prescription for therapy, but when she told me they would not actually put in the request for a referral, I knew I would not be going to therapy. I had been in that position before—taking one doctor's prescription to another to get a referral on behalf of the prescribing doctor. I know how confusing it is for a second doctor to interpret the prescribing doctor's intentions, diagnosis, and prognosis. More importantly, I knew how confusing it gets for my insurance company, especially if the doctor's confusion causes her to enter the referral request incorrectly. So, if he was not going to make the referral request for something *he* wanted me to do, I wasn't going to do it. I left his office, and as you can guess by now, I never returned.

From there the pain intensified. To make it even worse, the plantar fasciitis in my feet was growing worse. So, I was dealing with pain and inflammation in my right shoulder and both of my feet at the same time.

I sought prayer in my church's small group. I personally prayed and cried out to God continually. The pain only worsened. I had to quit going to church. It was a 30-minute drive, and by the time I got to service my feet hurt so badly I couldn't get out of the car or walk into the building.

One day, when I was making that trek back from Acworth to my home in Snellville, I had it out with God. I didn't know why He wasn't healing me, or why my search for a good doctor kept coming to dead ends. I did know that I was hurting and had lost all hope of ever feeling anything but pain.

My prayer started simply enough, "God, I am asking You, again, to heal me. The pain has become unbearable. Your Word says we are healed by Jesus's stripes, and I believe that."

From there, I got angrier and screamed, "I don't understand why You aren't healing me. I don't even know why I should believe You heal if You aren't going to. Seriously, why should I bother believing You do something, if You won't do it?"

I am not usually one to speak to God that way, nor do I condone doing so. But, I also know God is a "big boy." He is strong enough and big enough to handle our moments of anger. In His death on the cross, He bore all our pains and infirmities. He knows the human body and mind can only handle so much, and our expressing, even in anger, that we have reached our limitations does not anger Him or turn Him against us.

Unfortunately, it doesn't help us, either. I felt pretty guilty about getting so angry with the God I know loves me, but the pain had pushed me to the point that I had to get it all out, no matter whom it was aimed at. And I figured aiming it at God in that moment was better than risking the irreparable damage that could be done releasing that same pain and anger on another human being.

My help from God would come, even if it took a little longer than I would have liked.

In the fall of 2014, Lee finally joined all of us in Georgia. He was officially separating from the Air Force in January 2015, but because of the leave he had accumulated, along with leave that is typically granted for those preparing to retire, he was able to leave Joint Base McGuire-Dix-Lakehurst several months early.

I was glad to have him home with me. I was dealing with the pain from so many things, and I knew if another surgery became necessary, I wanted him with me.

Early in 2015 my right shoulder had gotten so bad that I knew I could not give up on my pursuit to find an orthopedist who would help me. I once again pored over the list of specialists in my network. I selected Dr. Davis and asked my doctor for the referral.

I was apprehensive about going to the new doctor, given all my previous experiences. But, the pain had increased to the point I couldn't move. I couldn't get dressed, and, if I did, I couldn't change clothes. This meant shopping for the clothes I needed as a new business owner was not an option. I still couldn't sleep on my right side because, if I did, I couldn't move at all in the morning. I would have to lie there until my body from neck to waist agreed to do what my brain instructed. I was miserable, and I didn't know what I was going to do if Dr. Davis turned out to be the jerk the previous doctor was.

Dr. Davis was actually the godsend I had hoped and waited for.

His staff was friendly and the waiting room was large and well-lit. Even better, they didn't keep me waiting for an obscene amount of time. I immediately felt at ease, and I was glad I had chosen him to be my doctor.

In the exam room, Dr. Davis nearly stole my heart!

We talked a little bit—the average things, about my condition, what I did for a living, where I was having pain, how bad it was, etc. The one thing that set Dr. Davis apart was what he didn't do. He did not put me through all the range of motion and strength tests. He gave me one test. That was all it took. He put his hands on my shoulder and forearm. He raised my arm to shoulder height and bent my elbow, bringing my hand toward my chest. He held my arm in that 90-degree angle for just a second and then pressed ever so gently on my wrist, pushing my hand toward the floor.

The pain nearly made me jump off the table, and for a fraction of a second I actually thought I might punch him.

His diagnosis was immediate. "You have some bursitis going on," Dr. Davis said. "Just a minute. I'll be right back."

He left the room and came back with what looked like a needle in his hand. I couldn't tell for sure; I was still reeling from the pain he had just inflicted.

"Turn a little and face the window," Dr. Davis instructed. I did so, and he sat behind me to my right. "I am going to give you a little shot of cortisone, and it should clear this right up."

"No, please don't," I said. I may have even whined or sounded like I was begging.

Dr. Davis did the most wondrous thing! He stopped and put his hands down. He sat on his stool, rolled back a little, looked up at me, and asked, "Okay. Why not"?

"Because they don't work for me. I mean, it will for a couple of days, and then it's like I never had it at all."

"And you already had the surgery on your left shoulder?"

"Yes."

"You had good results from that?"

"Yes, I did, and I have already been through physical therapy for the right shoulder twice."

When he was satisfied that surgery was my best option, Dr. Davis shrugged his shoulders and said, "Well, if you've already been through the wringer, we certainly don't want to put you through it again."

I felt the light of understanding brighten my entire countenance.

My help had come, at least for my shoulder, at last!

Dr. Davis walked me out to his scheduler. The surgery was set for April 15, 2015. The surgery and physical therapy went very well, and I knew that I had found my Earth Angel. I made a firm decision—Dr. Davis would perform all my future surgeries.

And, he has.

The Mental Attack

Shortly after Dr. Davis operated on my right shoulder, I started attending a church close to home. I hoped that going somewhere only ten minutes from home would be more bearable than the previous church I had attended. It did help, for a while.

The church I chose to attend only sang two songs on Sunday mornings. I could stand to worship during those ten minutes, but bending my ankles enough to sit down once the song service ended was quite painful. One morning, as I sat in my seat, someone needed to get past me to get to her seat farther into the row. She accidentally bumped my foot. It was the slightest touch, but it hurt so badly I literally came out of my chair. That was the final straw. I was going to see Dr. Davis again as quickly as I could.

Dr. Davis was not as quick to jump into operating on my feet as he was my shoulder. He, like all the other doctors, put me through the non-surgical "wringer." He first tried an ankle brace that was supposed to relieve heel spur pain. The brace was black neoprene and looked like something you might wear when you have a sprained ankle. The difference was that the heel had a donut-ring cushion. I can only assume the heel bone is supposed to sit in the center of the donut ring so that the cushion can keep the heel off the ground, which would understandably keep your weight off the pressure point and thus relieve your heel spur pain. Only it didn't. I stepped off the table onto the floor with the ankle brace on. The pain was so bad I think I touched the floor a whole quarter of a second before I jumped back on the examining table. These cushions obviously would not be the answer.

Dr. Davis and his team decided to make custom orthotics to see if they would help. These, unlike the first pair I bought, wouldn't cost me anything, and they wouldn't be cheap carpet foam, either. They would be the real deal, molded perfectly to my feet. Dr. Davis was sure the custom orthotics would relieve my pain, because unlike the lieutenant from many years before, he pointed out I have great arches; they aren't actually fallen at all. This is why finding doctors who will look beyond the "textbook" and see each patient as an individual is important.

The one thing that made these custom shoe inserts just like all the others was that they didn't work. I combined them with the sneakers Dr. Davis suggested I get. His exact words concerning the very expensive shoes that could only be found at The Running Store were, "They're ugly as sin, but they're the best."

I went to the store and bought a purple pair of shoes with orange trim. They weren't really ugly; they just didn't match anything I would ever wear. They were pretty comfortable, and made walking slightly more tolerable, but I was still in pain. In fact, I would like to mention the shoes' brand name is Hoka. They have changed their styles to be more attractive over the years, and they have shoes for every lifestyle, from standing to running to hiking. If you experience pain in your feet, I recommend you give them a try. They are expensive, but if your issue is simple and not as severe as mine, they are worth the money you will spend.

Dr. Davis finally knew what I had known for years—surgery was my only option if I was ever going to have any pain relief in my feet.

We scheduled the surgery for my right foot September 25, 2015. The only complication came from a slight infection in the incision. The incision site hurt so badly I had to take the bandage off and look at it, only to discover it was infected. The stitches had already been removed, and most of the wound had healed, but a small pocket at the edge of the scar had not. A ten-day round of antibiotics, and the infection cleared up without any further problems.

I did not rush to schedule the surgery for my left foot. I knew I would probably request it, but I really wanted to see if I could go without it. You never know what God will do, and I wanted to see what would happen if I waited.

When I finally relented, I went to see Dr. Davis about operating on the left foot. I honestly did not want to go through with it. A lot of fear had built up in me by then. Joan Rivers, who was well known for many things, not the least of which was too many plastic surgeries, had died. They say she had been put under general anesthesia one too many times, and it finally killed her. In light of her death, the fear of being put to sleep again attacked me in a way I can only describe as demonic.

The devil didn't stop there. My mind was attacked in another way. I will readily admit I used to watch too many crime shows, both real-life crime documentaries and dramas such as *Law and Order*. I had viewed too many stories about people making others sick or even poisoning themselves in order to gain the sympathy of others. It is an affliction known as Munchausen (when you make yourself sick) or Munchausen by proxy (when you intentionally make someone else sick). My mind was tormented with the fear that the reason God wasn't healing me was that I secretly liked all the attention of doctors and hospitals, and I somehow *wanted* to be in pain.

It was with the weight of this fear and guilt that I went into Dr. Davis's office to discuss the plantar fascia surgery on my left foot.

Dr. Davis looked at me. "Are you ready for the second foot," he asked.

I shook my head, "No, I'm not, really." I was suddenly more sheepish than I would be on an average day. I was just growing weary.

"No, but the pain is just too much," he said.

"Yes," I nodded, "it really is."

We continued to talk and I told him I had seen two rheumatologists about the possibility of my having something called polymyalgia, an autoimmune disease that keeps the muscles and tendons from recovering as quickly or as well as they should. The doctors had both told me I didn't have it. They both confirmed I had systemic inflammation, but neither could tell me why. To this day, I still have no answers as to why my body doesn't like to heal after an injury or why it builds up bone spurs the way it does.

Dr. Davis's response was nearly magical, though, as he looked at me and said, "Oh, you *definitely* have something rheumatological going on. Doctors just don't know what it is yet because rheumatology is a relatively new field of medicine."

I almost cried in relief.

"I could seriously hug you for that right now," I said as I told him how I had begun to secretly think there was something wrong with my mental health.

He grinned, shook his head, and assured me I was not crazy.

We set the surgery for March 30, 2016.

Again, the surgery went well. There was no infection this time, and one six-week round of physical therapy was all I needed. The long-term recovery was a bit slower than all my other surgeries. In fact, the scar on my left foot still swells and hurts if I am on my feet for extremely long periods of time, such as walking around Six Flags or the zoo. But, I can finally do daily activities like walking nature trails or cleaning the house without wishing I could get my feet amputated. Any relief compared to that is a blessing indeed!

I can never thank Dr. Davis enough for his help. I did see him later for some recurrent upper thigh pain, but after physical therapy didn't help and the MRI showed nothing was there, Dr. Davis decided medicine was not the answer. He put me on what is known as an anti-inflammatory diet—no grains, sugar, or legumes. The pain cleared up in a couple of months, and to this day, I can quickly feel the increased joint pain when I deviate from the diet's restrictions.

God knew I needed Dr. Davis. He knew the mental torment I was to face, and indeed was facing at the time, and that it would take a man like Dr. Davis to calm my fears and give me the assurance I needed to continue on.

The Pain Returns

About a year after Dr. Davis performed surgery on my right shoulder, just about the time my second foot was operated on, the pain in my right shoulder began to return. It wasn't too bad at first. Since it had taken a year for my left shoulder to fully recover and no longer have pain, I was willing to wait and see what happened. If the pain got much worse, I would go back to Dr. Davis. If it got better, there was no need to worry my doctors or myself again.

An incident in the fall of 2016 gave me a hint that I might need to brace myself for another wild round of doctors, surgeries, and physical therapy. Lee and I were walking on a wooded trail when we came to a very steep (nearly 90 degrees), two-foot tall incline. I instinctively reached out my right hand and grabbed the nearest tree trunk to pull myself up the tiny hill. I felt the same sharp and sudden pain I had felt way back when I first hurt my left shoulder all those years before on the job site. Only this time it hurt much worse. I couldn't move. I stood on the trail screaming with pain while Lee held me close. I eventually got myself together and we moved on.

I didn't think too much of the incident after that. But the pain in that right shoulder did continue to worsen.

By March 2017, the pain in my right shoulder was so bad I was forced to return to Dr. Davis. Once again, my shoulder had lost range of motion. I couldn't sleep on it, and I couldn't lift my hand or arm to a reasonable height.

Dr. Davis ordered another MRI. My follow-up appointment to go over the results was on a Wednesday. This time Dr. Davis referred to the arthritis the test showed in my distal clavicle, or outer end of my collar bone. He said he wanted to redo the surgery. This time, though, it would not be arthroscopy, with small, practically invisible incisions. No, he wanted to do an open surgery. He planned to remove more of the bone spurs and take out the arthritic part of my collar bone. We initially scheduled the surgery for the soonest that was available for both him and me—my birthday. Having surgery on my brother's birthday once was one thing, but no one wants surgery on her *own* birthday!

I left his office quite disappointed, but I was willing to go through anything I had to in order to get rid of the pain. When I got in my car I made a few declarations.

"I don't *want* to lose part of my clavicle," I said.

I don't know a lot about the human body, but I know that the collar bone gives your torso structure. It helps you maintain your posture, and I knew without it I could lose a lot of the strength and progress that had already been made with my shoulder as a whole. No, I did not want to go through with the surgery, but I did not see another option in that moment.

On Saturday, just a few days after my appointment with Dr. Davis, I went to a ministers' conference. I answered the call for prayer. The woman did not pray over me as much as she tried to prophesy I would have a son. But, to me, the important thing was that I knew what I went to the front for, and that was the answer I was intent on getting.

So, on Sunday, I went to the altar for prayer at my own church.

Bruce was available so I stepped up in front of him.

When he was done praying, Bruce looked at me and said, "God wants to give you a whole new shoulder. Not just repair that one. A whole new one."

By Monday, I was pain free enough that I called Dr. Davis's office and cancelled the surgery. But, the story doesn't stop there.

By Thursday the pain was beginning to return. It wasn't a very strong pain. It was just enough to let me know that it could come back if it really wanted to. That night, as I turned off the living room lamp to go to bed, I voiced my concerns to God. It occurred to me that plenty of people who love and trust God never receive healing.

I said, "God, who am I to expect healing without surgery when so many others never receive healing at all? Joni Eareckson Tada is still in a wheelchair after all these years. What makes me so different? Who am I that I should believe for healing?"

I believe God whispered to me, "You are still the little girl who, when the doctor told her she would have to have her tonsils removed if she got strep throat one more time, she said, 'Then I'll never get it again,' and you didn't. If you refuse to accept this surgery, you aren't going to need to have it."

I said, "Then I refuse to have it. I will not accept the need for surgery."

The pain left my shoulder instantly and, except for the typical pain that comes when I over-exert myself or start exercising it in ways I didn't before, the pain has not returned.

No matter what you go through—physically, spiritually, emotionally—God has an answer. It may take finding a different doctor, a doctor you would never think of seeking out. I never knew an orthopedist would provide answers to most of my difficult health questions, restore my mental health, and be the catalyst I needed to pray for a miracle in my shoulder.

I also never knew a gastroenterologist would prove to be the greatest counselor I would ever see.

The Answer
I Never Expected

The story I have written for this chapter is one I don't like to tell. It is the most embarrassing because of the symptoms I experienced. And, when you are addressing a public audience, you never know how someone is going to react to talk of anuses and bleeding. But, it just might be the one I believe to be most crucial, because it is the type of story *no* one wants to talk about if they can help it. I hope that telling my story will help others find the healing that eludes them.

I don't know exactly when the symptoms started. I do know I suffered for about 15 years before I was finally healed. As with all the other ailments, I went to many doctors. Like my many podiatrists, every gastroenterologist (GI) I saw wanted to start with the same test or treatment. And, like all my podiatrists, every GI was wrong.

I first went to the doctor with anal bleeding and soreness when we lived in North Carolina, though I can't remember the year. The bleeding was not constant, only when I had a bowel movement. The doctor said I had anal fissures and referred me to the GI, who wanted to do a colonoscopy right away to confirm there wasn't an underlying cause, such as polyps or cancer.

My friend Mary, the same one who had been there with me when I needed a ride to the clinic for my headache, took me to the hospital for the test. She told me the doctor came into the room while I was still asleep and told her there was nothing noticeably wrong.

"Then why all the bleeding?" she asked.

"Maybe irritable bowel," he shrugged, and rushed back out of the room.

Mary thought the doctor's attitude was very off-putting. He never talked to me after that, at least not that I remember, and I did not bother making a follow-up appointment with him. Irritable bowel is very treatable, and there are many medicinal options, but at that time it was still a diagnosis some doctors gave when they didn't really have a true diagnosis of what was wrong with you. If he didn't know what was wrong, there was not much need for me to see him again.

As with all my other aches and pains, I waited a couple of years before going to the doctor again about the bleeding.

This time, the new GI wanted to perform something called a sigmoidoscopy. He explained it was to look at the sigmoid, which was not quite as far up the digestive tract as the colon. Again, he found nothing wrong. Again, I would continue to do my best to keep the symptoms at bay (a feat that was truly impossible since I didn't know what caused them), and after several years I decided again to pursue some help.

I decided I did not want to try to see a GI after we moved to New Jersey. I was going to try something new, so I found a good internal medicine doctor. I went to the base medical clinic and got the appropriate referral. My efforts to try something new nearly became my undoing.

The internist, Dr. Maxim, was very nice, and he didn't rush to ordering a colonoscopy. I realize, though, in looking back on my conversations with him, that he had the same bad habit of mistaken assumptions that was characteristic of almost every other doctor I had seen.

Dr. Maxim assumed that my anal bleeding was due to the typical things, such as lack of fiber or straining to have a bowel movement.

"You don't have fissures," he stated confidently.

"Oh, really?"

"No, you have bleeding hemorrhoids. The blood is bright red, not black, so we know it is from outside of the body, or very low in the digestive tract."

My mind quickly flashed to a show I watched as a child called *Just the Ten of Us*, a spin-off of *Growing Pains*. It was a show about a family of ten—two parents and eight girls. The father was a girls' basketball coach at a high school. In the specific episode that came to mind, the father had to take leave from coaching because he needed surgery on his hemorrhoids. I didn't want surgery on my anus. The doctor's mention of it brought to mind the man in the sitcom laying on his belly on a stack of pillows after his surgery. I didn't need to worry too much about the surgery. Dr. Maxim had another option.

"You have a couple of options," the doctor broke into my thoughts. "You can have the surgery, or you can get Botox injections."

My mind quickly thought of some of the things I knew about Botox injections. I remember I had heard or read it was a way of relieving migraines. I also remembered an episode of *Frasier* in which Niles's injections kept him from blinking.

Dr. Maxim quickly explained what the two options meant.

"If you go through with the surgery, we go in and cut the sphincter muscle, which will make those bowel movements a lot easier. The downside is that you could experience incontinence."

Well, that is not an option! "And what about the shots?"

"The Botox shots will also help your muscles relax. We would hope it would allow the muscles to be trained before the shot wears off."

"But then, when the shots do wear off, I have to deal with the problem coming back, right?"

"Right," he confirmed, "you would run the risk of the symptoms returning. There is a possibility of incontinence with the shots, too."

"Okay," I said, "I will go home and think about it and let you know."

I did go home and think about it. My decision was that I wasn't going to go through with either option. Neither one sounded good. It would be several more years, but I would eventually learn how smart my decision to keep my distance from Dr. Maxim really was.

As time went on my symptoms worsened. There were times a bowel movement would make me so tired I actually had to take a nap. Sometimes having a bowel movement felt like a knife had been stuck up my anus and twisted. One time I was standing in the craft store when the need to go to the bathroom hit me. I knew by the way my entire gut, from my anus up into my hips, ceased up that the bowel movement was going to be difficult. Fortunately, at times like this I could get myself through the pain fairly drama-free. Other times, when I was at home, the pain from a bowel movement was so bad that I screamed out loud. A time or two there was so much blood in the toilet after a bowel movement that the water was opaque, with not even a slight amount of clarity. It was honestly quite scary.

What made all of this worse was that there was nothing consistent about my pain or my symptoms. Every time I thought

I had nailed a trigger, like corn or oatmeal, I seemed to react to a completely different food. All the foods doctors said should help, like vegetables high in fiber, only worsened my symptoms. I was completely perplexed, and quickly wearied of going from doctor to doctor each time the symptoms came back after a brief reprieve.

Soon, I found myself asking to see another GI. A new symptom had developed. I had been going to aerobics classes at The Y. The class went outside and jogged to the new fitness trail in Burlington, New Jersey. We stopped at one of the stations on the trail and did some squats. During the walk back to the gym, I felt a burning I didn't remember *ever* feeling. I was anxious to get to the ladies' locker room and find out what was going on. I was shocked at what I found. My underwear was soaked in blood, as if something had ripped open or ruptured. In spite of my doubt in a doctor's ability to help me, I had to try.

This new GI, like the others before him, wanted to do a colonoscopy. It is apparently the default test of all GIs when you are a new patient and your only symptom is bleeding during bowel movements. This doctor, like the two before him, discovered there were no obvious reasons for the bleeding. I didn't know where to go.

My Air Force doctor and I had a talk. I had done some research on the difference between irritable bowel syndrome and irritable bowel disease. He agreed with me on two points. The first was that it was more likely I had irritable bowel disease than that I had the syndrome. We also thought it was possible that I had endometriosis since the anal pain and bleeding worsened during my monthly cycle. He sent me to a gynecologist.

Fortunately, or unfortunately, Dr. Shipley, the gynecologist, agreed to the possibility of endometriosis. I had read that it is possible for endometrial tissue to attach to anywhere in the body, including the brain, and we were going to determine if this was the case. The unfortunate part is that his agreement meant I was going to have to go through yet another colonoscopy. This time, while I was on my cycle.

As you can imagine, I had another "failed" test. There was nothing showing on the colonoscopy. Nothing was wrong with my anus, my colon, or my uterus. I was back to square one. I was also back to a place of waiting until the time was right to seek out effective medical treatment.

In 2017 my breakthrough came.

The symptoms, which I had learned to keep at bay by avoiding corn and limiting my gluten intake, had come back yet again.

I asked to be sent to yet another GI. I didn't want to, but I was determined I was going to get to the bottom of my symptoms and find their root cause if it was the last thing I did, as the saying goes.

My doctor sent me to someone she thought would be perfect. That doctor didn't have any appointments readily available, so I had to see another member of the group. After I hung up with the very kind and helpful receptionist I looked online to do a little research on the doctor I was going to see. There were four reviews on him. That's it. And they were split 50/50—two good ones and two bad ones. They weren't just differing opinions on "good" and "bad," either. They completely countered each other. One negative review said Dr. Moore didn't seem to care or give them the attention they wanted. One positive review said just the opposite, that he was very attentive and took great care in listening to his patients' concerns. I decided to go ahead with the appointment. I would see him and decide for myself whether he was a good doctor.

The morning of my appointment, my very unpredictable symptoms came through for me. It is always easier to tell a doctor what is going on if you have the symptoms before or during the appointment. Otherwise, it's like taking your car into the shop for a noise that goes away every time you pull into the mechanic's driveway. You can describe it, but if it isn't happening in the moment the mechanic looks at it, you may be going back and forth until he can determine what the problem is.

Since I didn't know what to expect, and there was not much else I could do, I prayed on my way to Dr. Moore's office. "Lord, I don't know what to expect from this doctor, but I have decided to go ahead and see him. I ask that you give him wisdom in treating me, and that he will say *exactly* what I need to hear."

Dr. Moore was a lot like Dr. Davis. He sat and talked to me a bit. I gave him my history, telling him how long I had the problem, how many colonoscopies I had been through, and the occasional increase in anal bleeding to the point of making the toilet water opaque.

Dr. Moore had me get undressed and lie on the table so he could perform the usual exam. It hurt more than any other GI exam had ever hurt.

As Dr. Moore finished he said, "Okay, get dressed. I'll be back in a minute and we'll talk."

When he returned, he sat in a chair across from me and we talked a little more.

"Well," he said, "there is nothing wrong with you."

"Really," I asked in disbelief.

"No. There's nothing there. No polyps, no fissures, and no hemorrhoids. Nothing."

"Well, that's good. As long as I don't have go through another colonoscopy." I looked him square in the eyes, "I'm not having another one."

"No, you don't have to," he shook his head.

"Well, that's good. But, what about the symptoms? I was just bleeding this morning, before I got here. And you see nothing?"

Dr. Moore shook his head, "There's nothing there."

"Okay, then what is it?"

He looked a little downcast as he said, "Well, now I have to ask you the embarrassing question."

"Okay," I said with a slight laugh in my voice. All I could think was that his face may have changed, but at least nothing else did. He still had the same voice and body language. I remained completely at ease.

"Have you ever been raped?" asked Dr. Moore.

"Yes," I answered honestly, and without hesitation.

Although the minute details of rape are embarrassing to talk about, answering such a simple question honestly for a doctor I am comfortable with doesn't really embarrass me much at all.

"That's your problem," he said with complete confidence.

A very surprised, "Oh," was all I could manage.

He continued, "I mean, it's not my specialty or anything, but I have been reading a lot of articles about women who have all had the same symptoms you have, but nothing was wrong with them. The one thing they all had in common was that they had been raped. You need to see a psychiatrist."

We continued to talk. I don't remember what I said to him, but I made it clear somehow that I would not see a psychiatrist, preferring instead to see a Christian counselor.

"That makes sense," I told him. "I once suffered with pain in my hip for eight years. I finally went and talked with my pastor and received healing through forgiveness."

"Just see whatever type of counselor you are comfortable with."

"I can do that."

Dr. Moore looked at me with the most logical answer, "If you know it works, why would you not do it? If you have already experienced healing through counseling, and nothing else you have tried has worked, and someone tells you once again that counseling is the answer, it would only make sense that you would try it."

"You're right," I said. "I will find someone to see."

We talked some more and then Dr. Moore said, "But, you aren't having anal sex now, right?"

Now that *is the embarrassing question,* I thought.

"No," I shook my head.

I didn't think to tell him I have never had anal sex. Not once—not when I was raped, not willingly, not at any time. No, sex and my symptoms had no link in that regard.

When I got home, I was thrilled to know there was nothing wrong with me. At least not physically. Maybe I could finally quit unnecessarily seeing doctors over and over again for the same problem. I went into my office to call a couple of friends and tell them about my experience with Dr. Moore. First, I prayed.

"God, I know there are great counselors. Dr. Moore says I need to see one, and I did ask You to give him the wisdom to know what my answer was. But, I am very picky about the kind of counselor I will see. It would have to be a biblical counselor, and I don't know one in the area yet. Your Word says the Holy Spirit is our Counselor. So, until I find the right one, I will let Him be my Counselor."

I called my friends Gayle and Aris. I told each of them everything Dr. Moore had said and everything I had decided about letting the Holy Spirit be my Counselor. After all, I told them, all a counselor does is listen; they don't really offer any advice or instruction. The Holy Spirit can listen to me anytime I want, and He won't charge me anything or make me do weird things like imagery or memory alterations.

My friends agreed with me and were happy that I had found an answer. I have learned something more since that day, too. Since the Holy Spirit is indeed my Counselor, and He is always with me, He hears me every time I speak. I am healed a little more every time I tell my story. Meaning, the symptoms continue to diminish and the number of foods I can eat without irritation or bleeding increases. The symptoms don't even increase during my monthly cycle like they used to.

I have learned I can even eat corn again! I can't eat a lot of it, but at least I no longer have to feel deprived of it, and I don't have to worry about it accidentally being an ingredient in dishes when I eat out or go to someone's home.

I am grateful for everything God has done for me. All of the healings are a wonderful testimony of His great love for us. Even when the healing wasn't miraculous, or took a while to manifest, God was there guiding me to the right doctors. I will forever give Him praise for all He has done and continues to do for me.

Healing Comes
in God's Presence

Just when I thought the previous chapter was going to be the last one, God revealed He had other plans. There was one more healing I needed to go through. It is just one of the many ways God heals, but I hadn't experienced it in its purest form yet—simply being in God's presence.

This story will be different from the others I have shared. I am not going to tell you all of the details, but just enough that the story makes sense. I have even removed most of the names, except where citing a source is required and proper. This story is intended to focus only on the events, and when you read it you will understand why.

There was a certain condition I had for many years. The symptoms showed up when I was in a car for very long, when I exercised, and when I slept. Although I had the condition for a horribly long time, I didn't pursue an answer like I did with other medical conditions. I did go to a specialist once. They hooked me up to a machine and did a special test to see what was occurring inside my body when the symptoms were present. But, of course, like taking your car in for a "noise," the symptoms didn't occur once during the test. Because the symptoms didn't appear, the doctor conducting the test didn't find anything wrong.

The symptoms even went away for a while after that test. They didn't stay gone for long, though, and I learned to live with them because they weren't "that bad," and probably were even a little "normal." By 2018 the symptoms had worsened to the point that I could barely stand them or myself.

In September 2018 I went to a women's retreat. I had known about the guest speaker for almost 20 years after I first saw her and her husband speak at a church I attended in Fayetteville, North Carolina. This retreat was the first time I got to officially meet her face to face. She and I sat in her room and had a wonderful "girl chat" about the presence of God and His goodness and life. Out of that conversation came my request to be mentored by her, something I had wanted since I first heard her speak. She said yes! She wasn't sure how it would work with our living on opposite sides of the country, but I assured her it would work somehow.

One of the things I have always admired about this woman is the amount of time she spends in God's presence. I wanted more than anything to learn to enjoy His presence for myself the way she does. I had no idea where or how to start, but I was determined to find out once I got home. Being in her secret Facebook group for mentoring would surely help. I trusted God to show me the rest.

Shortly after the retreat my church, Influencers Church, had their annual conference. That weekend, during the conference, my symptoms from this particular condition were so bad that I couldn't stand it anymore. By Sunday I was sore and in pain, and was losing hope that I would ever be healed. During worship that morning, I told God I couldn't take it anymore, that I wanted to be healed of this condition once and for all.

During the sermon, I pondered this book being released. After all, except for this chapter all the writing had been done. I was anxious to get it into the hands of people who could benefit from it. But, the thought came to me that if I released the book too soon, healing from this particular condition would come after the book was already out.

That's okay, I thought. *If the healing comes afterward I can always print a revised or updated version.*

In my spirit I heard, "Do you want to be healed badly enough to wait to release your book so this healing can be included in it?"

I said, "Yes, Lord, I can wait."

I didn't know how long I would have to wait. I didn't know what I would be doing while I waited. But, I was sure God said wait, so I resolved in that moment that I could wait and trust God that His timing would be perfect. Here's the best part—in just a matter of minutes God was going to tell me what I would be doing in my waiting.

Daniel Kolenda was the conference speaker who had stayed over to preach our service Sunday. As Kolenda closed out his message, I headed to the foyer where I served as a volunteer in event registrations, but as I got to the door I was compelled to stop and finish listening. He was talking about the story of Daniel in the lions' den. Kolenda told us that when Daniel comes out of the den, all he says is that God's presence was with him and that the mouths of the lions were closed. The point was that too often we tell stories of what God has done, but give our problems all the "glory." We tell all about our sickness, our symptoms, our pain, our addiction, our crimes, and leave only a tiny bit of time in the story to tell what God has done to deliver us. Even though we give God credit, the power of what He has done gets lost in all of the tragedy of our story.

Kolenda pointed out we need to focus more on God's presence and what He has done. We, like the prophet Daniel, should give

God the glory He deserves more often and simply say, "All I know is I spent time in God's presence and He saved me."

I knew in that moment what God wanted. I realized all the other stories in this book were exactly what Kolenda had described—they told all about my tragedies and how angry I was with God and doctors. God wanted something different for this last story. He wanted me to be healed in His presence. He wanted me to include it in this book so others would know He can and is willing to do it for them, too. He wanted to be sure He got *all* the glory and that, unlike my other stories, His presence would be the main focal point.

But, I walked out of the sanctuary that morning not knowing any more than I did before about *how* to actively live in the presence of God. I still didn't know what waiting for my healing was going to look like. I didn't know how many days or months I would have to live in God's presence. I didn't know how much time each day I was going to have to spend in prayer for it to be considered "in His presence." I didn't know if my focused prayer time was going to include prayer and Bible reading, worship, or some other activity. I *did* know that once I figured out what I had to do, I was going to do it with my whole heart.

About a month after Influencer's conference, I started getting sick. I would get sick for a week or two, get better for a week, and then get sick again. This lasted from the end of November through March. It was starting to affect my life and impact my ministry in the church. I had to stay home a lot of Sundays and missed a lot of Wednesday Bible studies.

One Bible study leader called me to talk about my being sick so often. She explained that she saw great leadership potential in me, but that if I was going to walk in my calling, I couldn't keep getting waylaid by every sinus issue or flu that came my way. There were times during those few months that I was truly very sick. There were other times, if I am honest, I have to admit I just used not being well as an excuse to avoid small group just because I was so comfortable staying at home and not going anywhere. This leader and I discussed how, no matter how insignificant *I* see my role, when I am absent from the group, it affects everyone.

The leader didn't want to leave me where I was. No, she wanted to mentor me into "greatness" (her word, not mine). I agreed to submit to the mentoring process, knowing it was what I needed. I had to learn to be stronger in soul and spirit so I could be stronger physically. I had never had a successful mentorship, so I was a little apprehensive, but I also knew she only wanted what was best for me. She took a different approach to mentoring than any I had heard. She said being a mentor was about talking to me and finding out what my needs were and then helping me get those needs met.

I told my leader about my encounter with the speaker at the women's retreat in September and of what I believed God told me concerning this final healing story coming from His presence. But, I told her the one thing I needed most was discipline in my Bible reading and prayer life. I had served God most of my life, but had never developed a consistent, daily prayer and Bible reading habit. I would try, but then stop when I got busy or bored with whatever study guide I was using. I had started and stopped so many Bible reading plans that I had given up using them. I knew, though, that if I was going to learn to spend time in God's presence, this was the place to start.

My newfound mentor knew firsthand conditions and supposedly "magical" steps people have often put on prayer. I have heard most of them. Things like, "Leave time in your Bible reading for God to speak to you about what you just read." "Prayer is a dialogue, not a monologue. Get up in time to pray and then be quiet. You have to allow time for God to converse with you." There are many more, but you get the point. I had tried devotionals and journaling. I had tried listening to the Bible on cassette or CD instead of reading it, which didn't work because I would get distracted and never hear what was said.

The solution to all of my questions and problems turned out to be quite simple. My mentor told me to start small, with just ten minutes—five minutes each—in prayer and Bible reading. She told me to set a timer and not to pressure myself to do more. I could go over, but I didn't have to feel obligated to pray or read longer if I didn't want to. This was supposed to be completely pressure-free. I did that for a week, and every day for that week, she held me accountable, calling or texting to encourage me to keep up the progress I was making. The second week we changed it to 20 minutes total.

By the third week my mentor quit checking on me daily and changed to once every few days to once a week, allowing me to now be a "spiritual adult," responsible for my own growth. Her plan worked, and now I have no problem spending as much time in God's presence in prayer and reading as I want each day. Sometimes it is as long as 90 minutes. Other times it is only 20. It is always up to me and God and the burdens I take on in prayer that day. Never, though, do I feel like I must be in God's presence a certain way or for a specific amount of time. I know that even when I am not sitting still in God's presence I carry His Spirit, and thus His presence, with me everywhere I go. It is a *lifestyle*, not a brief event relegated to only the time I set aside each day. God doesn't want any of us to confine His presence to brief, or long, encounters that we then forget as we go about the rest of our day. No, He wants us all to live in His presence every moment of every day, in all that we do and say.

In April 2019 I went to see the speaker from September's retreat again. She was ministering in Morganton, North Carolina. That Saturday was to be a full day set aside for prayer for our nation. The speaker does some teaching, and there is a lot of worship, but our purpose is to really pray. We pray for wisdom for government leaders, school safety, returning prodigals, and for many more topics, 30 in all.

Morganton is a four-hour drive from home which meant I had a lot of time to worship and pray in the solitude of my car. Having never forgotten what I believed was God's promise about my healing coming from His presence, this was one of the things I requested.

"God, I just want to come out of this weekend healed after spending time in Your presence," I prayed.

Ordinarily the symptoms from the medical condition I was battling would be quite evident after such a long drive. The trip to Morganton was no different. I arrived at my hotel Friday night with my symptoms clearly present, and in full force, I might add. I forgot about my prayer in the car, though, as I went through the entire day Saturday completely focused on praying, worshiping, and spending time in God's presence. I stayed for the church's Sunday morning service, again focusing on worshiping God and not anything else I wanted from Him.

The drive home Sunday was different. For the first time in years my symptoms did not appear once while I was driving. Prior to that weekend I felt blessed if I made it through a 30-minute drive without my symptoms appearing, but here I had now made it four hours without a single symptom.

It was entirely the presence of God. No one prayed for me, except for the little bit I privately said Friday. No one laid hands on me or prophesied my healing. God did it, just as He promised, because I had learned to live in and trust in the power of His presence.

Not every healing has come to me miraculously. In fact, as I write this I am preparing for another surgery. This will be my seventh one, a redo on the surgery originally done on my left shoulder.

But, God wanted this story included so you know that when you need healing, you must *start* with His presence. It was one of the last things I learned to do, but you can, and should, make it your first. If you need an accountability partner or a mentor to help you learn to make God's presence a lifestyle, actively seek for one and pray that God will lead you to the right person or persons. Then, you too can share the wonder of your story, that however God chooses to heal you, miraculously or not, He gets all the glory. The pain and suffering you went through will not be the focal point of your story. The presence, power, and glory of God will be your testimony.

Developing a Peaceful Heart and Healthy Body

A large part of this book was written based on Proverbs 14:30, but there are many more verses we can look at regarding a peaceful heart and a healthy body.

"A joyful heart is good medicine, but a broken spirit dries up the bones" (Prov. 17:22).

"Therefore, confess your sins to one another, and pray for one another so that you may be healed. The effective prayer of a righteous man can accomplish much" (James 5:16).

"Beloved, I pray that in all respects you may prosper and be in good health, just as your soul prospers" (3 John 1:2).

You can tell from my stories that some of my healings came when I let go of hurt, resentment, or bitterness. It is interesting that all of these are varying degrees of each other.

When I was looking for answers to the pain and problems in my body, it was choosing to be at peace that led me to the right doctors, like Dr. Davis.

When I finally said, "God, I don't know why You aren't healing me. I don't know why I don't heal from injuries without subsequent surgeries. But, I am willing to submit to Your plan for me, no matter what is. I accept that it's just who I am," was when God would finally led me to the right doctor.

Even when my guidance didn't come right away, taking such a humble posture in my prayers gave me the peace I needed so that I could find the best way to get my body healthy. It was really quite freeing.

I know there are those who are going to read my story and be healed. They are going to find the will to forgive those who hurt them and unexplained, relentless pain is going to finally leave their bodies. Some are going to summon the will and strength to keep pressing on to find the right doctor or medical treatment. Some will be inspired to be healed miraculously, as I was on more than one occasion. Others may never get healed in a way that physically manifests itself, but their hearts (their souls) can be at peace and their bodies be healthy in other ways.

I mentioned Joni Eareckson Tada in one of the chapters. I only know a small part of her story. Tada was paralyzed as a teenager in a diving accident. She was taken to many pastors and preachers. Still, she was not healed. She was made to feel she just didn't have enough faith, and was almost shamed into giving up on God and herself, thinking it might be her fault she remained in a wheelchair.

I don't remember what finally turned Tada around and caused her to trust God. And I don't want to speak for her, either.

But, I want to tell you what I see and hear when she speaks. I see the joy of a woman who has a peaceful heart. She prospers in her soul, and for that reason she prospers in life. Many would say she is not healed, so her body isn't "prospering." I don't believe that, though. Of course, I don't know all the health and medical issues associated with being a quadriplegic. But, from what I see in following Tada's life and ministry over recent years, she gets around quite well. She travels around the world and speaks to vast audiences. She spreads God's love to others. Her faith in

Him inspires others to believe in Christ as their Savior. She runs a camp for disabled, or "other abled," children each summer, and collects wheelchairs for those in need. I would say that is being quite prosperous "in her body" as she does what God has called her to do. Tada's body effectively does what it can while she is on Earth. One day, she will shed her earthly body and walk on streets of gold. For now, she simply lives the best life she can through God who gives her the ability to do so.

The reasons why don't matter. It does not build anyone's faith to constantly ask God why healing never comes, or why healing doesn't come in the way or manner we want it to. It didn't do me any good. It didn't build my faith when I searched for a year for answers on why my body often tests positive for systemic inflammation, yet the doctors can't find a medical reason for it. It only made me miserable to continue searching for an answer that wasn't there.

Dear reader, please learn to trust that God has an answer for you. He wants to get it to you. You just have to be willing to accept it and to listen for it. Don't assume how it will come. It may come through a doctor or a mentor, or directly from God to you.

Cheryl Salem was recently speaking with an intimate group of women about her daughter, Gabrielle, going to heaven. The family prayed. Friends prayed. Pastors prayed. Gabrielle prayed. As far as Gabrielle was concerned, she simply was not going to die, and, as Salem says, "She didn't."

Salem reminded us that when Gabrielle died, she didn't really die. All Gabrielle did was shed her earthly body by walking right out of it and stepping into heaven. The Salem family could have wasted a lot of time trying to understand *why* God allowed Gabrielle to leave them at such a young age. But, the why doesn't matter. Knowing why on this side of heaven won't change anything. It won't ease our suffering. It won't help us move on. It won't inspire others so they can find healing after a loss.

During her time on Earth, Gabrielle's soul prospered because she believed in a God who loved her, who wanted what was best for her, and who would allow only what was best for her. Her body eventually prospered, too, because it is now completely whole and free of pain and sickness. And now, sharing her story in a way that allows God to heal them and others is one of the many ways the souls of the Salem family prosper.

If they spent their time wallowing in self-pity or devoted their time to finding out why, they would be of no use to anyone on Earth. God could never use them, and as long as they were in their earthly bodies, their in-body experiences would be less than prosperous.

But, because they have peaceful hearts that trust God in everything, and maybe even in spite of some things, they have healthy bodies. They are individually healthy, of course, but there is more.

Their ministry is a "body," a physical manifestation of the work God is doing throughout the world. Their family is a "body," a cohesive unit of people who live, love, and work together within their own family and in the lives of others. The list of healthy bodies, groups of people, the Salems have formed go on. I don't know that I could truly list them all because I only know a snippet of their lives. I do know that I have been blessed by them in ways I couldn't be if they didn't choose to have peaceful hearts and healthy bodies that reach out and share the joy and love of God with others.

Beloved, whatever health or physical ailments you face today, please know that God is with you. If you have not received the work His Son did on the cross, start there. From there, allow the Spirit of God to bring His peace into your heart so that you can have a healthy body. Trust that not every person will be the "vision of perfect health" often implied when people teach on healing. But, our bodies can be healthy in the way that allows God to best utilize us for His glory all the days of our lives.

Peaceful Heart Coaching

Many people find that like Michelle they have
unexplained pains or illnesses.

These same people have had at least one traumatic
event in their lives that no one else knows about.

It is time to break the silence and voice those things
no one else has ever heard.
Or maybe you did speak up once, and no one believed you.

There is someone who believes you, and someone who will be a
safe place for you to tell your story.

There is someone who will help you let go of the emotions that
have held you back, made you sick, or caused you pain.

Book your call with Michelle Watson to see if her storytelling
coaching is right for you.
Visit www.thecharmingartist.com/booking today.

About the Author

Michelle Watson is the President and CEO of Topflight Communication, Inc. and an Artisan Storyteller at The Charming Artist.

She was born in Springfield, Missouri, but she has always considered Enid, Oklahoma, where she spent most of her childhood, to be her hometown.

Michelle obtained her B.A. in Communication Studies at Regent University in 2012. She graduated with honors and was a member of Lambda Pi Eta, the National Communication Association's official honor society.

A lifelong lover of words, Michelle is an editor, a writer, and a speaker, who practices the art of putting words together to create masterpieces. Writing is just one of the many art forms Michelle uses to tell stories. As a fiber artist she knits, quilts, and embroiders. On canvas she produces mixed media and acrylic paintings. Michelle also studies piano, and plays the flute and clarinet.

Michelle's books focus on topics of interest to Christians and business owners. Her books are the subjects of speeches and keynote addresses that entertain Michelle's audiences while giving them helpful information and pathways to healing through submission to God. Her speaking topics include Christian Inspiration, Overcoming Obstacles, and Self-Editing Techniques.

Although she is not much of an outdoors person, she does enjoy hiking trails with her husband and mountain vacations.

Michelle and her husband live in Snellville, Georgia. They have one daughter, one granddaughter, and one grandson.

www.ingramcontent.com/pod-product-compliance
Lightning Source LLC
Chambersburg PA
CBHW052046270326
41931CB00012B/2646